PERGAMON BIO-MEDICAL SCIENCES SERIES

Editor: Roger Maickel
Indiana University
Bloomington

The Meaning of Human Nutrition
PBMSS-2

GW00693811

The Meaning of Human Nutrition

Mina W. Lamb
and
Margarette L. Harden
Dept. of Food & Nutrition
College of Home Economics
Texas Tech University

PERGAMON PRESS INC.

New York · Toronto
Oxford · Sydney

PERGAMON PRESS INC.
Maxwell House, Fairview Park, Elsmford, N.Y. 10523

PERGAMON OF CANADA LTD.
207 Queen's Quay West, Toronto 117, Ontario

PERGAMON PRESS LTD.
Headington Hill Hall, Oxford

PERGAMON PRESS (AUST.) PTY. LTD.
Rushcutter's Bay, Sydney, N.S.W.

Library of Congress Cataloging in Publication Data

Lamb, Mina Marie (Wolf) 1910–
    The meaning of human nutrition.

    (Pergamon bio-medical sciences series, 2)
    Bibliography: p.
    1. Nutrition. I. Harden, Margarette L., joint
author. II. Title. III. Series. [DNLM: 1. Nutri-
tion. QU 145 L218m 1973]
RA784.L34 1973   613.2   72-11636
ISBN 0-08-017078-1
ISBN 0-08-017079-X (pbk)

Section 10 contributed by
DR ILSE H. WOLF
Professor of Home Management and Consumer Economics
Department of Home and Family Life
College of Home Economics
Texas Tech University

Illustrations by
REAL MUSGRAVE and DICK CHEATHAM

Printed in the United States of America

Second Printing

Contents

Preface

This book is designed as a textbook to present the core of information basic to human nutrition. Students must use references to develop deeper knowledge and understanding. This book directs learners to include activities meaningful in the development of their behavioral concepts about nutrition.

An effort is made to relate food and human nutrition to the history of man's struggle for survival and to efforts to control the environment to his advantage. Several lists of events are included to relate these efforts chronologically in history to show how great discoveries or ideas have evolved gradually.

Each section includes "Objectives" designed for student achievement, some information and explanation of pertinent ideas in nutrition, a list of suggested "Activities for Student Learning," and an "Inventory of Knowledge" which students can use to test their comprehension of each section. "Activities for Learning" are planned for students to explore and apply the factual information in several different ways in order to develop particular concepts about nutrition; these are not included as a device for the professor to use in grading student comprehension. The format of this book is designed to encourage students to implement the objectives by means of personally selected behavioral responses to recommended food consumption practices. Hopefully, this approach will encourage the learner to practice recommended dietary patterns before he tries to direct others to do so.

MINA W. LAMB
MARGARETTE L. HARDEN

About the Authors

Mina W. Lamb (Ph.D., Columbia University) is Margaret W. Weeks Professor, College of Home Economics, Texas Tech University, Lubbock, Texas. Since 1933 Dr. Lamb has been active in teaching and research in the fields of nutrition, home economics, public health, and general education. She is a member of several professional associations, is listed in *"Leaders in American Science," "Who's Who of American Women"* and *"Who's Who in American Education"* and is the author or co-author of nearly forty articles which have appeared in various professional journals since 1937. In 1965, named outstanding Professor in Texas, Dr. Lamb was the recipient of the Minnie Stevens Piper Professorship from the Minnie Stevens Piper Foundation.

Margarette L. Harden (M.Sc., Texas Technological University) is Assistant Professor, College of Home Economics, Texas Tech University, Lubbock, Texas and directs her own dietetic consulting service for small hospitals and nursing homes in the western Texas area. Since 1967 Ms. Harden has been active in research, teaching, and study in the fields of nutrition, home economics, and plant proteins. She is a member of several professional societies, has published numerous articles and abstracts in professional journals, and is the producer of three audiovisual programs: *"Food Made the Difference," "Animal Research in Nutrition Education,"* and *"Your Food — Chance or Choice."*

1

The Study
of Nutrition

**What Basic
Preparations Need to
be Made for the Study
of Human Nutrition?**
A student in pursuit of knowledge about any given subject should be well informed about the publications produced for such a study. The current explosion of knowledge makes a list of references from journals almost obsolete before the printing is completed. Nonetheless, the generally accepted books of any one period should be available to the conscientious student.

Some books are timeless in their value and need to be part of the educational background of a student who undoubtedly will want to include such publications in a personal professional library.

A teacher would guide students to evaluate books to select for a specific need at any given time.

OVERVIEW OF THE STUDY OF HUMAN NUTRITION

From early childhood, people are taught that the basic physical needs of man are food, shelter, and clothing. Since the beginning of recorded history, man has struggled desperately to acquire enough to eat. History records a select few who indulged heavily in consumption of excessive food (e.g., King Henry VIII), but the mass of humanity has been highly concerned with "filling its stomach," not questioning whether the food had a purpose or a function as long as it relieved hunger. Only since 1890 to 1910 has the function of food been given serious consideration by men in research and medicine. Since 1910 they

1

have been trying to describe a "recommended diet" for a long healthy life. Much confusion has reigned in the struggle to define an adequate diet, as is illustrated by Ronald Deutsch in his book entitled *Nuts Among the Berries*, by Frederick J. Simoons in *Eat Not This Flesh*, and by Gerald Carson in the illustrated history of "patent medicines" entitled *One for a Man and Two for a Horse* and in his *Cornflake Crusade*. Other authors have conveyed the complexity of man's concern for food in such books as *The American and His Food* by Richard O. Cummings, *The Geography of Hunger* by Josue' De Castro, *Attack on Starvation* by Norman W. Desrosier, and *The Ecology of Malnutrition* by Jacques M. May. Prominent among all these treatises is *A History of Nutrition* by E. V. McCollum which further reflects the fact that man had great difficulty in clearly defining an "adequate diet." Man long has been confused about what to eat. However, only recently through economic prosperity and abundant agricultural production of food in the United States have the majority of people had a choice in what to eat. As a result food fads, quackery, and unwise food selections have increasingly become a major concern of those who are abreast of research and are genuinely concerned about human health.

Few discoveries in medicine have been met with wider acclaim than the revelation that certain components in foods markedly improve man's ability to live longer and to perform more effectively. Most people believe their state of health from day to day depends on what they eat. Few people realize the profound effect of the afferent stimuli to the brain from the sensory reaction to sight, smell, touch, and taste of the food. Conditioning and learning are also important to the acceptance of foods. Diets vary with cultures, races, nations, and even with regions and the seasons of the year, but nutrition is universal.

Nutrition is the result of dietary practices after foods have been eaten, digested, and nutrients are absorbed into the blood. Nutrition is the science of nourishing the body—the food that is eaten and the way that the body uses it! Graham Lusk in 1906 at Physiological Laboratory, Cornell University Medical College and the Russell Sage Institute of Pathology in his classic treatise, *The Science of Nutrition* gave this definition: "Nutrition may be defined as the sum of the processes concerned with growth, maintenance and repair of the living body as a whole or of its constituent organs." These processes include the chain of events whereby the nutrients obtained from food reach the individual cells where they are used for energy, built into the cellular structure, or become constituents of compounds performing a regulatory function. Thus the nutrients in food are those chemical components of the food that perform one of three roles in the body: to supply energy, to regulate body processes, or to promote the growth and repair of body tissue. All people throughout life have need for the same nutrients but in different amounts. Therefore, the body is the product of nutrition; heredity provides the blueprint for the body, and nutrition supplies the building materials.

LAYMAN'S VIEW OF PHYSIOLOGICAL FUNCTIONS OF FOOD

GO POWER:	To supply energy, furnished by carbohydrates, fats and proteins, and regulated by vitamins and mineral elements.
GROW POWER:	To build and maintain cells, tissues and organs, furnished by water, protein, vitamins, minerals, and energy.
GLOW POWER:	To regulate body processes for energy and maintenance, furnished by all nutrients coordinated and functioning together.

In its broadest sense, the subject of nutrition is concerned with those physiological functions of the body related to the nutritive constituents of foods and to a chain of events whereby these constituents become available for utilization by the cells. Elimination of wastes and the regulatory mechanisms of the body must be considered as a part of the nutritional processes.

In discussions on the nutritive needs of the body, the terms diet, food, foodstuff, and nutrient have been used. These terms are sometimes used synonymously; foodstuff was the original term to refer to the constituent substances of food and had essentially the same meaning as nutrient in current usage. Natural foods usually contain more than one nutrient; for example, analysis shows that milk is composed of water, protein, fat, carbohydrate, mineral salts, and vitamins. On the other hand, food extracted from natural agricultural products may be pure, as for example, oil from cottonseed or corn, starch from corn, sugar from beets or from the sap of sugar cane, and many others.

Nutrition now occupies an important place in a number of college and university curricula, including home economics, animal science, horticulture, medicine, and the allied health or paramedical fields. With the rapid advances in research, knowledge of nutrition is constantly expanded and new interpretations and applications are presented. The primary source of this expansion in knowledge of nutrition is in the pure sciences of chemistry and physics applied to biological structures and processes. An example of this type of research is that which resulted in the identification of the deoxyribonucleic acid (DNA) molecule identified as a key structure in heredity.

The science of nutrition is a relative youngster in the scientific field;

The American Institute of Nutrition was recognized as a distinct field in 1934. In order to anticipate the forward direction that research in nutrition may take, a backward review of the past is helpful.

Historical Background

Nutrition is a comparatively new member of the group of biological sciences. Hippocrates in 607 B.C., however, realized that certain foods were necessary for proper development of the body and recommended various diets for different conditions. Leonardo da Vinci presented definite ideas about food along with his work as an artist, sculptor, inventor, and designer of a submarine.

The date of the actual conception of nutrition can be placed in the latter part of the eighteenth century when the great French chemist, Antoine Laurent Lavoisier in 1783, produced experimental evidence that the heat of the animal body is derived from the oxidation of carbon and hydrogen similar to the process utilized in a flame. Lavoisier and the French physicist, Laplace, put guinea pigs in a chamber surrounded by ice and from the amount of ice melted in a certain period of time, they measured the heat given off by the animals. A determination of the oxygen consumed and the carbon dioxide produced by these animals showed that only 81% of the oxygen combined with hydrogen to form water. A calculation of the heat produced by oxidation of both the carbon and hydrogen gave figures very close to those obtained with the ice calorimeter.

Lavoisier next attempted to apply the results of his observations to a human subject, using an associate, Seguin. A drawing made from memory by Mme Lavoisier after the death of her husband in 1794 shows Seguin breathing through a mask into a series of globes, which afforded a means for determining the oxygen consumed and the carbon dioxide exhaled. The exact method of the experiments is unknown since Lavoisier was executed by the Paris Commune before he was able to publish his results in full. Fortunately, an abstract of this work was published which sets forth conclusions so fundamental to the development of a knowledge of nutritional processes as to earn for Lavoisier the right to be regarded as the Father of the Science of Nutrition.

The French physiologist, Francois Magendie (1783–1855) was the first to differentiate among the food constituents and evaluate them experimentally through animal studies. The modern viewpoint that several kinds of nutritive substances are necessary was set forth by

William Prout (1785–1850) in a book published in 1834. He divided the food nutrients into the saccharine group, the oleaginous group, and the albuminous group for which we now use the terms carbohydrates, fats, and proteins. Eight years later the great German chemist, von Liebig (1803–1873), published the results of his critical studies in which he showed that these "organic foodstuffs" are oxidized in the body.

Liebig's initiation of modern methods of organic analysis paved the way for extensive work in food analysis and the analysis of urine, feces, and body tissues and thus made possible the investigation of metabolic changes. Liebig recognized the fact that protein contains nitrogen and suggested as early as 1842 that the nitrogen of the urine might be used as a measure of the protein destruction in the body. This method was later demonstrated by Bidder and Schmidt and was established by the German physiologist, Carl Voit (1831–1908).

At the close of the nineteenth century (1895), the American scientist Atwater (1844–1907), who had studied under Voit published a summary on the analyses of foods, emphasizing nutritive ingredients (in terms of carbohydrates, fat, and protein), digestibility, fuel value and the ratios between nutritive values and costs. Atwater considered it poor economy to purchase fruits, fresh vegetables, and eggs since cheaper foods would serve just as well in meeting nutritive needs, according to nutritional concepts of his time. Vitamins and most mineral elements had not been identified prior to 1910; their role in human nutrition was not even suspected. In discussing Atwater's work, McCollum said, "Atwater visualized the coming of a time when farmers should be able to consult tables showing the cost of protein and energy in various crops, and, taking into account digestibility of their food elements, to select the cheapest sources of these nutrients for compounding their rations for feeding animals. Fortunately for his peace of mind he never saw the effects of restricting animals or men to diets which might have been compounded on his advice. Also, it is very fortunate that housewives did not, so far as we are aware, attempt to follow his advice in the feeding of their families."

Of course the early nutritionists, such as Atwater with the U.S. Department of Agriculture, Armsby at Pennsylvania State University, and McCollum at Wisconsin State University, were primarily concerned with animals rather than with human beings. They were solving problems of great economic value to the frontier country which was just becoming scientifically oriented in its agriculture and industry at the turn of the century.

Benedict at the Carnegie Institute in Boston and DuBois at the Russel

Sage Foundation of Medical Research in New York, in 1910–1920 pursued concern for the importance of human nutrition by analyzing respiratory exchange as related to heat production in healthy, normal persons of different ages and in ill or abnormal persons. Except for modifications proposed by Boothby, Berkson, and Dunn of Mayo Clinic, Benedict's and DuBois' data still serve as the reference standard for prediction of basal energy expenditures.

The interest created in nutrition by the work of Atwater, Benedict, and others resulted in many dietary studies on people in different parts of the world who performed different kinds of work and were engaged in varied occupations. The findings in terms of energy as calories and as protein needs were used as a basis for establishing the dietary requirements of the human body.

At the beginning of the twentieth century, nitrogen balance was investigated by Henry Russel Chittenden of Yale University. As a result of his findings in prolonged experiments on different groups of men, he became an advocate of low levels of protein intake as being most conducive to health. Chittenden's work stimulated further study of the quantitative needs of man. Sherman's compilation of data from available nitrogen balance studies showed the minimum protein requirement to be close to the level advocated by Chittenden, but Sherman recommended that the daily allowance should provide a "margin of safety" which should be 50% above the minimum required for nitrogen equilibrium.

Sherman offered much leadership in the development of the currently emphasized Recommended Dietary Allowance of the Food and Nutrition Committee of the National Research Council. These allowances established in 1941 were expected to be revised at intervals as data from research indicated the need. Revisions have occurred periodically, the most recent being in 1968; a new one to be released in 1973.

The beginning of the twentieth century also saw the initiation of studies on the amino acid composition of proteins in relation to their nutritive value and the significance of individual amino acids in nutrition. Kossel, Fisher, and Osborne were pioneers in protein analysis. Willcock and Hopkins in England and Osborne and Mendel in this country were the first to establish the essential nature of certain amino acids. Their work has been extended with the employment of more highly refined methods by W. C. Rose and others. Shortages of the usual sources of high quality proteins created by World War II and the following years of exploding populations have stimulated renewed interest in foods and protein analysis as well as in all other aspects of nutrition.

Twentieth-century developments have included a greater recognition of the importance of the mineral elements in nutrition and the discovery and gradual elucidation of a large number of heterogeneous substances known as vitamins. The recognition of the chemical activity of vitamins as constituents of enzyme systems has greatly increased knowledge of their functions in metabolism and other chemistry of living tissue.

Areas of investigation which challenge the twentieth-century investigator are the interrelationships among nutrients and the control of nutritional processes. A better understanding of these factors will add other important chapters to the development of the science of nutrition.

The tools of nutrition investigation have closely followed developments in chemistry, biology, microbiology, and physics. An understanding of the chemistry of nutrients and their metabolic products was followed by investigations of the intermediary metabolites which have recently been greatly facilitated by the use of biological tracers in the form of radioactive elements.

The use of laboratory animals for research in nutrition has been and continues to be of incalculable value in the quest for knowledge. Currently improved techniques for human experimentation are beginning to furnish means of studying the applicability of the findings on laboratory animals to problems of human nutrition. Probably the most valuable of animal research projects have been those involving longevity studies. Increasing evidence indicates that the final evaluation of an adequate diet may need to be measured in the success of future generations and not alone in the current one. Such long-term projects are now underway with findings which are giving direction for human behavior.

Food and History in North America

As the population grew in a new area of the world such as that of the United States, people began to plan for food production and to store supplies, thus resulting in greater availability of food. Some regions and nations did not achieve increased food in proportion to increased people. There is no way of knowing the numbers of people who have died from malnutrition throughout history and who continue to do so today. In the United States prior to 1900 and even until 1940, scarcity of food in many regions and at certain times of the year was a chronic dilemma. The development of agriculture as a science and a business with the assistance of technology has assured today's people an abundance of high quality food. In the 1970s the problem is primarily one of choice of food; are we willing to choose and eat the food in amounts required for health?

References and Suggested Readings

Beeuwkes, A. M., Todhunter, E. N., and Wiegley, E. S. *Essays on History of Nutrition and Dietics.* Chicago: Amer. Dietet. Assoc., 1967.

Carson, G. *Cornflake Crusade.* New York: Rinehart, 1957.

Carson, G. *One for a Man and Two for a Horse.* New York: Doubleday, 1961.

Cummings, R. *The American and His Food.* Chicago: University of Chicago Press, 1940.

De Castro, J. *The Geography of Hunger.* Boston: Little, Brown & Co., 1950.

Desrosier, N. W. *Attack on Starvation.* Westport, Conn.: Avi., 1961.

Deutsch, R. *Nuts Among the Berries.* New York: Ballantine Books, 1962.

Holden, G. K., and Lamb, M. W. Early foods of the Southwest, *J. Amer. Dietet. Assoc.*, **40**, 218 (1962).

Lusk, G. *Clio Medica*, a series of primers on the history of medicine, X, *Nutrition.* New York: Hoeber, 1933.

May, J. M. *Studies in Medical Geography.* New York: Hafner, 1961–70.

Maynard, L. A. Early days of nutrition research in the United States of America, *Nutr. Abstr. Rev.*, **32**, 345 (1962).

McCollum, E. V. *A History of Nutrition.* Boston: Houghton Mifflin, 1957.

McCollum, E. V. From *Kansas Farm Boy to Scientist.* Lawrence, Kansas: University of Kansas Press, 1964.

Sebrell, W. H., Jr., Haggerty, J. J., and editors of *Life. Food & Nutrition.* New York: Life Magazine, Life Sci. Library, Time Inc., 1967.

Sherman, H. C. *The Nutritional Improvement of Life.* New York: Columbia University Press, 1950.

Simoons, F. J. *Eat Not This Flesh.* Madison: University of Wisconsin Press, 1961.

A symposium—Landmarks of a half century of nutrition research, *J. Nutr.* Suppl. 1, Part II, **91**, 2 (1967).

William O. Atwater—A Biographical sketch (1844–1907), *J. Nutr.*, **78**, 3 (1962).

TECHNICS TO ESTABLISH VALIDITY OF INFORMATION

Objectives

1. To identify a person as an authority and evaluate the reliability of the information dispersed in books, magazines, and other areas.
2. To compare the traditionally used technics of witch doctors, quacks, and charlatans to those in current use.
3. To recognize the recourse of an individual who receives misinformation by mail, is approached by illicit salesmen, or identifies questionable food or food handling.
4. To differentiate fact from fallacy since publishers do not necessarily assume this responsibility in their publications.

What Basic Preparations Need to be Made for the Study of Human Nutrition?

Students of each decade face an ever increasing array of publications about any given subject. In addition to current publications on nutrition, certain books continue to contribute to the basic core of knowledge. One problem unique to the area of nutrition and other medical and health topics, is the need to establish validity in publications. Students must recognize the criteria by which to validate a publication. Some general guidelines to be used in the evaluation of books are:

1. Examine the preface of a book to determine its purpose and scope.
2. Identify the author as to educational background, employment, experiences, and major contribution (if identified). Be wary of unidentified authors or those of vague but superlative backgrounds.
3. Determine outstanding and unique features of the book which may include chapter organization, annotated tables and graphs, pertinent pictures, and references.
4. Scrutinize the information, references, data and authorities used in the publication.

Burns states that both professional and lay people need help to distinguish valid publications from those which are questionable. An excellent evaluation of books about nutrition is presented in a bulletin which identifies bases for making decisions concerning the validity of a publication:

> (Burns, Marjorie, Nutrition Books: *A Guide to Their Reliability*, Ithaca, N.Y., Cornell Extension Bulletin 1158, Revised, 1967.)
> 1. The dietary recommendations in the book are not compatible with the formation of sensible food habits.
> 2. The contents of the book are misleading due to the selective use of facts to support a biased or unwarranted conclusion without presenting an adequate and objective review of the topic under consideration.
> 3. Opinions and recommendations in the book are at variance with those of the majority of nationally recognized nutrition authorities.
> 4. The book contains little or no information that is scientifically factual.

A student of nutrition has many decisions to make involving interpretation of opinions voiced or written about food and its function in health and well-being. The following lists of criteria are designed to assist in arriving at valid decisions.

Criteria to Validate Scientific Information and Data

1. Statistical methods are used to determine variability or central tendencies of results.
2. Reproducible results are those which have been or can be replicated by other researchers and are used to check data and concepts.
3. Controlled experiments are designed to establish the limits of research; i.e., a positive control group in an animal feeding study is used to show the optimum or maximum response; the experimental groups are used to show response to various levels of substance or food in question in contrast to a negative control which shows the lowest level of performance.
4. When using live animals, these must be pure-bred, environmentally controlled animals in order to assure a standard experimental design and reduce unpredictable variables. Such animals have been standardized to achieve results which can be replicated.

Criteria to Validate the Authority of a Speaker, Author, or Disperser

1. Who is the informer? By whom employed? Where? Educational background for the topic discussed? What else has been said by this person? Has the material written by him been published? Where?
2. Where was the report made and to whom — laity or professional? Was it oral or written? Was it clearly and succinctly stated? Are there advantages of printed information over that given orally?
3. Whose references were used? Was the name and place of publication included? Did he use quotations or did he interpret "freely" the results of other researchers or writers?
4. Were data included? Were these validated by including number of cases, range of results, the control of variables? Were conclusions based on data presented?
5. Who was the publisher and where is it located? What sales promotion accompanied the publication? What was the purpose in publication?
6. What financial interests were involved? Are products offered for sale? Who profits from the promotional pitch?

Analysis of Faddism

Patterns of wishful thinking which lead to support of quacks can include the following:

1. A tiny grain of truth can snow-ball into a mound of fallacy.
2. Man believes he can accomplish wonders if he is given a magic token.
3. All human beings hope for a miracle to occur; all people believe in magic, even if just a little.
4. Surely someday, somewhere, somehow each person can get something for nothing; e.g., she hopes that she can get results without paying the price; she wishes that she could get a slim figure without self-denial at the snack bar.

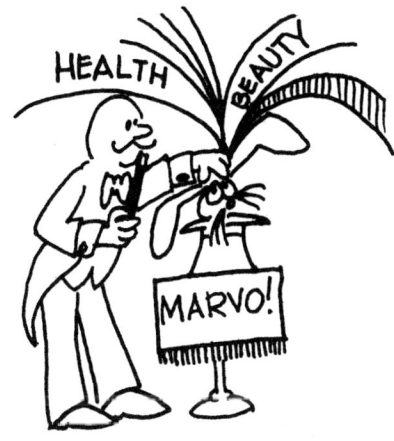

Fig. 1.1 All people believe in magic, even if just a little.

5. The hope never wanes that one example is proof for a broad generalization, even when the example was misinterpreted by an untrained person who did not relate cause and effect correctly.
6. People are prone to look for an "easy way out" of a perplexing or tedious situation, i.e., the need to lose excess body fat.
7. People in all ethnic groups have some family-propagated customs, superstitions, and concepts of cause and effect which are not based on rational judgment; e.g., Uncle George was sick the night that he ate fish with milk for supper.
8. After years of privation and limited food supplies, people have acquired the concept that "if a little bit is good, a lot is better for you"; e.g., the diet supplement is the best one to buy whenever it has multiple times the National Research Council's Recommended Dietary Allowance for a given nutrient.
9. Individuals are susceptible to sales pressures; misleading or false advertising causes many a "victim" to purchase expensive, unneeded novelty foods, diet supplements, cooking or food preparation devices with a sense of false security.
10. Basically the reason that people accept false and misleading information, illogical data, and fraudulent devices is a lack of knowledge about the human body—its structure and function, and about food—its composition and role in human nutrition.

Types of Common Fads Which Appeal to Many Persons

1. Some beauty aids promise to make the hair and skin more acceptable or youthful in a short period of time.
2. Devices or diet supplements are advertised to improve the muscularity or physique of an individual whether it be for the biceps, breast development, or virility.
3. Many "things" are promoted as cure-alls for multiple conditions of ill health, e.g., vitamin pills and protein tablets used as substitutes for faulty diets.
4. "A bad-tasting, noxious food, or odd substance undoubtedly must be good for you" is an idea probably developed during the days of witch doctors and sorcery. Often the quality of America's abundant inexpensive food is questioned and degraded in order to establish the need for a supplement.
5. Weight reduction schemes, pills, devices, and propaganda promise immediate results in producing "Twiggy-type" figures in people of different genetic heritage.
6. Constant appeal to the American emphasis on youth with the consequent fear of aging and loss of virility causes many persons to grab hastily at gimmics, pills, and diets in a vain effort to avoid the inevitable.
7. In the 1970s the major confusion centers around "organic foods," their virtues and advantages over those produced by use of chemical fertilizers, insecticides, and other innovations of technology. Obviously all plant and animal products are composed of organic molecules as contrasted to inorganic ones. Basically nothing is wrong with "organically grown" food and neither is there with conventionally grown and processed food. Gardening is an excellent hobby and healthful recreation; it does not lend itself for production of the commercial quantities at prices that most consumers can afford to pay. To buy and eat "organic food" is a luxury which only a few eccentric individuals can afford.
8. Research in food and diet fads has indicated that faddism is prevalent among more affluent and educated consumers who can afford the cost of their fanaticism. In this affluent group are youth who make use of organic food and vegetarian diets in their efforts to establish an identity and as a protest against the "establishment."

Are Fads Bad? Definitely True!

1. Money that may be needed for the basic necessities of life is wasted on items hastily chosen by emotionally guided decisions.
2. No benefits are obtained from fads; in fact, certain practices and pills can be harmful, delay needed treatment, or use limited financial resources.
3. The real problem involved often is that people may tend to neglect a real health problem with which they are faced or treat a minor symptom and not the underlying cause.
4. Fad items are developed for quick, lucrative sale, and for impulse purchase. They are not based on a need that has been established by laboratory tests, weighing pros and cons, or even on a desire established by the purchaser.
5. False security may be gained by using fad diet supplements, e.g., a mother provides a useless dietary supplement to a child instead of a well-balanced meal.

Organizations to Supply Information and Guidance on Health Quackery

Inquiries can be directed to any of the following addresses:

1. American Medical Association, 535 North Dearborn Street, Chicago, Illinois 60610.
2. National Health Council, 1740 Broadway, New York, N.Y. 10019.
3. Food and Drug Administration, Department of Health, Education, and Welfare, Washington, D.C. 20204.
4. Post Office Department, Bureau of the Chief Postal Inspector, Washington, D.C. 20260.
5. American Cancer Society, Inc., 219 East 42nd Street, New York, N.Y. 10017.
6. The Arthritis Foundation, 1212 Avenue of the Americas, New York, N.Y. 10017.
7. Federal Trade Commission, Bureau of Deceptive Practices, Washington, D.C. 20580.
8. National Better Business Bureau, 230 Park Avenue, New York, N.Y. 10017.
9. The American Dietetic Association, 620 North Michigan Avenue, Chicago, Illinois 60611.
10. Consumers Union of U.S., Inc., 256 Washington St., Mount Vernon, N.Y. 10550.

Activities for Learning: To Validate Authors and Information

1. You should visit a pharmacy, health food store, or similar establishment and compare the variety of goods merchandised, price per package, size of container, and other information with those of foods commonly sold in grocery stores.
2. You may want to write to an organization that supplies information and data on health quackery to obtain current information.
3. Be sure to watch and study television commercials, news items, advertisements in magazines and newspapers in order to evaluate the validity of information presented.
4. A learning experience would be to role-play a situation in which classmates can recognize the interplay between the traditional technics of witch doctors, quacks, and modern charlatans and those of the innocent uninformed housewife who wants much but has limited resources and judgment.
5. You may work alone or with a partner to create an exhibit or poster demonstrating ways to validate an authority, information, or a product and to expose facts to a selected group of learners.
6. You need to evaluate manuscripts by both professional and questionable authors.
    (a) Select a manuscript from a reliable source and evaluate its characteristics.
    (b) Select a manuscript from a questionable authority and evaluate its claims and information.

Reference Books

General Nutrition

Bogert, L. J., Briggs, G. M., and Calloway, D. H. *Nutrition and Physical Fitness*, 9th ed. Philadelphia: Saunders, 1973.
Chaney, M. S., and Ross, M. L. *Nutrition*, 8th ed. Boston: Houghton Mifflin, 1971.
Fleck, H. C. *Introduction to Nutrition*, 2nd ed. New York: Macmillan, 1971.
Guthrie, H. A. *Introductory Nutrition*. St. Louis: Mosby, 1971.
McHenry, E. W. *Basic Nutrition*, rev. ed. Philadelphia: Lippincott, Nursing Division, 1963.
Mitchell, H. S., Rynberger, H. J., Anderson, L., and Debbie, M. V. *Cooper's Nutrition in Health and Disease*, 15th ed. Philadelphia: Lippincott, 1968.
Pike, R. E., and Brown, M. L. *Nutrition: An Integrated Approach*. New York: Wiley, 1967.
Robinson, C. H. *Proudfit-Robinson's Normal and Therapeutic Nutrition*. New York: Macmillan, 1969.
Taylor, C. M., and Pye, O. F. *Foundations of Nutrition*, 6th ed. New York: Macmillan, 1966.
Wilson, E. D., Fisher, K. H., and Fuqua, M. E. *Principles of Nutrition*, 6th ed. New York: Wiley, 1966.

Wohl, M. G., and Goodhart, R. S. *Modern Nutrition in Health and Disease*. Philadelphia: Lea & Febiger, 1970.
Williams, S. R. *Nutrition and Diet Therapy.* St. Louis: Mosby, 1969.

Food Composition

Church, C. F., and Church, H. N. *Food Values of Portions Commonly Used*, 10th ed. Philadelphia: Lippincott, 1970.
Nutritive Value of Foods, Home and Garden Bulletin No. 72. Washington, D.C.: USDA, 1964.
Watt, B. K., and Merrill, A. L. *Composition of Food, Raw, Processed, Prepared*, Agr. Handbook No. 8. Washington, D.C: USDA, 1963.

Supplementary Information

Agricultural Research Service. Food Intake and Nutritive Value of Diets of Men, Women, and Children in the United States, Spring 1965. A Preliminary Report, ARS 62-18. U.S. Department of Agriculture. Washington, D.C., 1969.
Barber, M. I. *History of the American Dietetic Association*. Philadelphia: Lippincott, 1959.
Deutsch, R. *The Family Guide to Better Food and Better Health*. Des Moines, Iowa: Meredith, 1971.
Eppright, E., Pattison, M., and Barbour, H. *Teaching Nutrition*, 3rd ed. Ames, Iowa: Iowa State College Press, 1967.
Heinz Handbook of Nutrition, 3rd ed. New York: McGraw-Hill, 1967.
Kruse, H. D. *Nutrition: Its Meaning, Scope and Significance*. Springfield, Ill.: Thomas, 1969.
Lowenberg, M., Todhunter, E. N., and Wilson, E. D. *Food and Man*. New York: Wiley, 1968.
Martin, E. A. *Robert's Nutrition Work with Children*, rev. ed. Chicago: University of Chicago Press, 1954.
McWilliams, M. *Nutrition for the Growing Years*. New York: Wiley, 1967.
Present Knowledge in Nutrition, 3rd ed. New York: The Nutr. Foundation, Inc., 1967.
Scrimshaw, N. S., and Gordon, J. E. *Malnutrition, Learning, and Behavior*. Cambridge, Mass.: M.I.T. Press, 1968.
Yearbook of Agriculture, Foods. Washington, D.C.: USDA, 1959.
Yearbook of Agriculture, Protecting Our Foods. Washington, D.C.: USDA, 1966.

2

Basic Concepts
About Human Nutrition

What Were Early Man's Concepts about Survival on Earth?

For centuries man's major efforts have been directed to securing food, shelter, and clothing for himself and the family. This concept has prevailed even until today. Man finally learned to produce food, to preserve it for storage, to process and package it for trade with others, and ultimately to supply food cherished by the majority of his ethnic group.

Throughout history, concepts about food and survival have been closely allied to those dealing with man's relationship to other men and to his environment. When man has abundance from which to choose, he requires knowledge on which to base his judgment in selection. A democratic government assumes increasing responsibilities for control of quality in food production, processing, and distribution. It becomes actively involved in human affairs to reduce the gap between the "haves and the have-nots" and to improve the total environment which handicaps people in achieving their genetic potential.

Thus nutrition education becomes a major goal in the education of people for a democratic society.

EARLY CONCEPTS ABOUT FOOD AND SURVIVAL

Objectives

1. To recognize man's concern for food throughout the centuries.
2. To relate man's dietary problems to technological changes.

The Ages of Man in Search for Food

The Forager

In the beginning, man lived as a forager in certain regions on earth, in the valleys and the plains where plants and animals were abundant. He depended on plants to furnish the mainstay of his diet and ate the herbivorous animals when he could catch and kill them. At times he even ate carnivora to tide him through a famine.

The Hunter

After an abundance of food was no longer available to forage, man became a hunter. He now learned how to throw a rock, how to shape the rock, and how to add a handle. Man probably migrated with the seasons and the weather as he hunted for food. As a hunter, man had leftovers

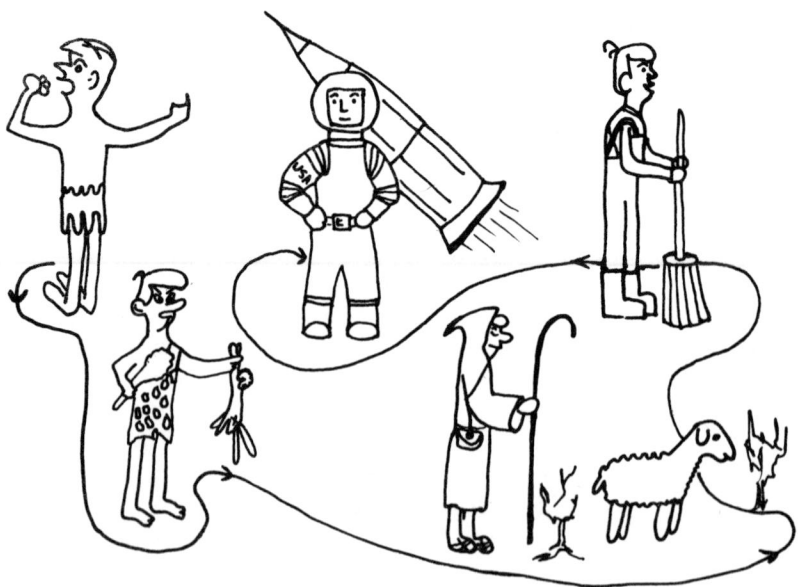

Fig. 2.1   The ages of man in search for food (Designed by Nancy Bell).

and produced by-products; he wore hides, entertained himself and his friends with horns, and decorated himself and his caves with various kinds of ornaments made from carcass remains. Undoubtedly the babies used strips of hides as "pacifiers" and for teething. What kind of daily dietary pattern did the hunter have? Either he stuffed with available food or he was hungry as he hunted for his meal.

The Agrarian

Gradually, man found spots on earth which were attractive and where he could survive if he remained the year around. With time, man created tools, collected and planted seeds for food production, and domesticated animals. "Manpower" was converted into "ox or horsepower."

The Industrialist

As people became industrially oriented, a derogatory viewpoint developed toward the agrarian. The agrarian was referred to as a peasant, "ein bauer" (German) or "peon" (Spanish): "the man with a hoe, the brother of the ox." Changed attitudes occurred in the United States only gradually after 1862 when the government created the Land Grant Colleges to educate the man and his wife in agriculture and home economics. Such long-range planning has promoted agriculture and home economics as professions and has helped to create an abundance of food and fiber for man.

The Scientific

This is the current epoch in the development of man. Tremendous strides in science occur daily in all aspects of life. One has only to pick up a newspaper, turn on the radio or television to gain new information. Yet, in this time of mass populations in urban centers many millions of people are malnourished. Never has there been a greater need for the application of science of nutrition.

The Humanitarian

All the science and resulting technology are for naught unless man learns to care about and to be concerned for his brother. This concept was proposed almost 2000 years ago and is slowly being accepted by people. Its ultimate acceptance by the governing majority is essential for man's survival on earth.

CURRENT BASIC CONCEPTS OF NUTRITION

Objectives

1. To define the origin of national concern about nutrition.
2. To identify government-sponsored efforts to improve the nutritional status of United States citizens.
3. To analyze the Basic Concepts of Nutrition as presented in 1967.
4. To derive sequential nutritional concepts to use in teaching at all levels.

National Nutrition Conferences

1941   The first National Nutrition Conference was called by President Franklin D. Roosevelt to consider the nutritional status of people in a nation at war. Results of physical examinations of conscriptees were shocking when half of the young men called up for military service were rejected because of one or more physical defects.

1952   The second conference convened to review progress in nutrition and to determine ways to strengthen existing programs.

1957   At this conference the chief concern was for the nutrition education of mothers; as well as for motivation of other family members to develop sound dietary practices.

1962   The emphasis at this conference was on nutrition education which would bring nutrition information to all people in the United States. It was realized that different technics would be required to reach and motivate people in various age groups to become concerned about their health and their dietary practices.

1967   This conference can be called the organizational conference because of the emphasis on representation from all those agencies and organizations related to the nutrition of people. The keynote of the conference was to call attention to the gap between the knowledge about food and nutrition and the practice of recommended dietary habits. Stress was placed on the need of each generation having to "be taught anew the proper habits of nutrition as a guide for good health" according to Mary M. Hill, nutritionist, Consumer and Food Economics Research Division of the USDA in the *Nutrition Program* News for May–June 1967.

1969   The White House Conference on Food, Nutrition, and Health was called by President Richard M. Nixon for December 2–4, 1969, and directed by Dr. Jean Mayer, professor of nutrition at Harvard University. It was probably the largest nutrition meeting ever held and was keynoted by Dr. Mayer's definition of hunger (1969–70).

An explanation of the feeling of the Conference is given in a summation entitled Dr. Mayer Defines Hunger to a Reporter, published in *Nutrition Today*, **4**: 7–16, 1969–70:

We're dealing with words that are taken by various people with meanings, all of which are legitimate but not exactly the same.

For the nutritionists, hunger means not enough food in terms of the total amount. Malnutrition means the wrong kind of food.

For most of the people engaged in social action, hunger has a broader meaning. It is synonymous with deprivation. Deprivation of food is one aspect, but deprivation of money, of social status, of right—all these things are also part of the overall picture.

Malnutrition itself has a vague meaning. It is a lot of things that are not being done for people that ought to be done. . .

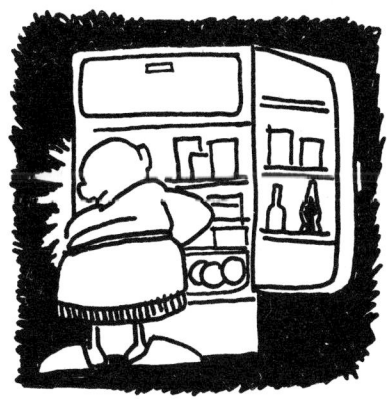

Fig. 2.2 Hunger has a broader meaning.

1971 The National Education Conference based on the theme: Youth-Nutrition-Community includes three objectives:
1. Look at youth today—his values, life-styles, eating habits, health.
2. Look at youth in his environment—physical, biological, social.
3. Identify effective ways of working with youth in providing support in the development of his food habits.

Implications were that youth is willing but nonetheless is the victim of many forces which detract and deter his concern for health and adequate dietary practices. Most of the stress forces on youth are products of the socioeconomic-political problems of society itself caught in the web of rapid change.

Basic Concepts in Nutrition

At the 1967 Nutrition Education Conference Dr. Ruth M. Leverton, Assistant Deputy Administrator of Agricultural Research Service, recalled the recommendation of the 1952 Conference that basic concepts of nutrition be formulated. A subcommittee of the Interagency Committee on Nutrition Education was appointed to formulate the concepts. The committee recognized "that concepts are the 'meanings' that direct a person's responses and decision." "Concepts of nutrition are as dynamic as the research findings on which they are based" and ". . . like the recommended dietary allowances and the food guide, concepts must be reviewed from time to time." According to Dr. Leverton, ". . . these basic concepts of nutrition for nutrition education can remain useful and dynamic during the decade ahead." These basic concepts are:

1. Nutrition is the food you eat and how the body uses it. We eat food to live, to grow, to keep healthy and well, and to get energy for work and play.
2. Food is made up of different nutrients needed for growth and health. All nutrients needed by the body are available through food. Many kinds and combinations of food can lead to a well-balanced diet. No food, by itself, has all the nutrients needed for full growth and health.

   Each nutrient has specific uses in the body.

   Most nutrients do their best work in the body when teamed with other nutrients.

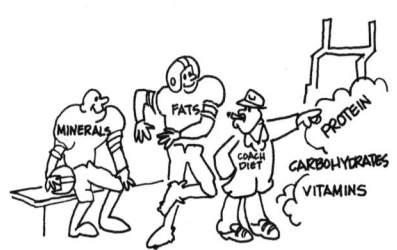

Fig. 2.3 Most nutrients do their best work when teamed with others.

3. All persons, throughout life, have need for the same nutrients, but in varying amounts.

   The amounts of nutrients needed are influenced by age, sex, size, activity, and state of health.

   Suggestions for the kinds and amounts of food needed are made by trained specialists.
4. The way food is handled influences the amount of nutrients in food, its safety, appearance, and taste.

   Handling means everything that happens to food while it is being grown, processed, stored, and prepared for eating.

Application of Concepts to Problem Situations

Surveys of attitudes of students toward nutrition show that they are bored with it, that it is "old hat," the same stuff over and over, year after year. Educators need to consider this criticism seriously and design a definite regular sequential learning. For example:

1. ability to identify different kinds of food as to physical appearance, taste, odor, forms in which commonly eaten, and its use in family meals and the school lunch;
2. ability to recognize functions of foods and their classification into food groups;
3. ability to comprehend that food functions in the body to achieve its physiological needs;
4. ability to analyze the role of food in meeting the needs of various people – physiologically, psychologically, and socially.

Progressive sequence for the development of a concept can be described in terms of a young child's response within a single term or semester of school, when he:

1. identifies food visually,
2. recognizes reasons for eating food,
3. accepts new food and realizes that he should taste it,
4. names different foods and the groups to which each belongs,
5. identifies ideas about why food is important to his health and growth,
6. discovers that other families, other groups of people have different food patterns.

The Interagency Committee on Nutrition Education (ICNE) which formulated the four basic concepts in nutrition described them as: "fundamental ideas to be developed through nutrition education, not facts to be presented or taught as such" and "the concepts will provide a springboard for program planning." Also, this committee reported that: "nutrition educators will need to keep in mind the process by which concepts are developed – the way people learn – when they select specific supporting principles, ideas, and facts related to concepts."

Some illustrations to support ramifications of the basic concepts for a professional level course in human nutrition designed for all home economists and related health personnel are:

Concept 1

Nutrition is the food you eat and how the body uses it:

• The energy needed for growth, maintenance, and bodily activity is provided for by the oxidation of nutrients.
• Inadequate, excessive, or imbalanced intakes of nutrients may be detrimental to health.

- Each nutrient has a physiological role and interrelationship with other nutrients in bodily functions.
- The physical and chemical properties of nutrients are related to their digestibility, absorption, and reactions in the metabolic processes.
- A variety of food is most apt to supply a balance of nutrients for human welfare.
- Food lends itself to scientific research and artistic expression as a commodity of universal concern.
- Both overnutrition and undernutrition can lead to undesirable results in the body.

Concept 2

Food is made up of different nutrients needed for growth and health:

- Food contains nutrients that are essential for human life: proteins, lipids, carbohydrates, minerals, vitamins, and water.
- Plant foods are increasingly necessary for populations in the continuing imbalance between arable land and increasing populations.
- Food sources of nutrients vary within cultures, sociological strata, geographical regions, and economic resources.
- A variety of food will supply the nutrients required by people in different geographic locales.
- The food guides are food groups based on the nutrient content.
- All nutrients need to be available from food at each meal to assure the most efficient utilization.

Concept 3

All persons, throughout life, have need for the same nutrients, but in varying amounts:

- Food habits and preferences are a complex interaction of physiological and psychological factors associated with food.
- Dietary inadequacies at crucial periods of growth can have permanent results on the growth and development of the organism.
- Physiological needs for food vary with the individual and are related to the metabolic functions characteristic of that age.
- Persons select food for nonnutritional and nutritional factors.
- Individuals of all ages are more likely to accept a wide variety of foods if they have variety in experiences, appreciation, and knowledge of food and if their environment reinforces positive attitudes.
- Physiological stress, i.e., infections, emotions, pregnancy, and levels

of physical activity influence the nutritional needs of the various age groups.
- National and international agencies cooperate in research and in assisting people of the world to have better diets through increased productivity, improved processing procedures, and greater dispersal of food supplies.
- Each person is the product of his life's nutritional sufficiency.

Concept 4

The way food is handled influences the amount of nutrients in the food, its safety, appearance, and taste:

- Unsupported and exaggerated claims related to dietary supplements of foods may result in the consumer spending money needlessly for these items.
- Research extends our understanding of and ability to control the nature of food and its behavior.
- The nutritive value, sensory quality, and safety of food may be altered by the physical and chemical environment.
- Rational choices of nutritional food products become more difficult as number and ways of merchandising food increase.
- Federal, state, and local agencies provide guidance by establishing standards for the consumer in purchasing food.
- The handling of food in the home is of vital concern in assuring maximum retention of nutrients and of palatable quality.

GOVERNMENTAL AND EDUCATIONAL INFLUENCES ON NUTRITION

Objectives

1. To interpret the role of government in a democratic society to sponsor education and well-being of all citizens.
2. To identify the sequence of regulations which permitted or delegated the establishment of educational institutions.
3. To translate current legislative regulations for the improvement of the health of all citizens in the United States.

Chronological Sequence of Governmental and Educational Influences on Nutrition

1787   Northwest Ordinance provided that "schools and the means of education shall be forever encouraged."

1791   Tenth Amendment of U.S. Constitution—reserved education to be administered by the states.
1803   Public lands given for education in Ohio.
1818   First money granted to the states for education by federal government.
1862   Land-grant colleges established by first Morrill Act.
1865   Freedman's Bureau created to assist in education of freed slaves.
1867   Department of Education created in federal government.
1869   Iowa State College recorded a course in "domestic economy" for women.
1871   Iowa State College listed courses entitled "Domestic Economy."
1873   Kansas began its "Domestic Economy" curriculum.
1874   Illinois developed a "systematic and thorough" program for women students.
1887   Hatch Act created Agricultural Experiment Stations.
1914   Smith-Lever Act established cooperative extension programs.
1917   Smith-Hughes Act provided federal assistance for vocational education.
1947   National School Lunch Program created by Congress in Department of USDA.
1948   Mundt law for global program in education approved by Congress.
1953   U.S. Office of Education was made a part of Department of Health, Education, and Welfare with the Secretary in the President's Cabinet.
1954   Segregation in public schools ruled unconstitutional by U.S. Supreme Court.
1960   Golden Anniversary White House Conference on Children and Youth called by the President.
1968   The Child Nutrition Act was passed.
1969   White House Conference on Food, Nutrition, and Health called to lay the foundation for a national nutrition policy and to create an awakened public opinion.

Current Legislative Regulations of Major Impact

Endorsement of Bread and Flour Enrichment by States

Since 1946, enrichment laws have been adopted by more than half the states. Today all "family flour" shipped in interstate trade is enriched. Authorities estimate that 80–90% of all bread and macaroni foods are enriched. Crackers and other cereal products are enriched or fortified

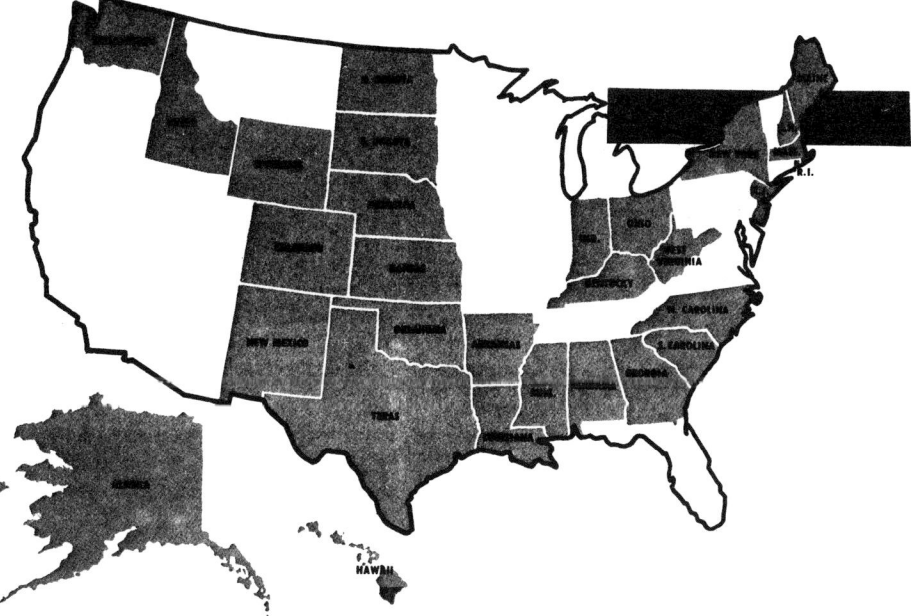

Fig. 2.4 The 30 states designated on this map and Puerto Rico passed enrichment laws prior to March 1965. (Reproduced by permission of The American Institute of Baking.)

at the decision of the processor and more brands are carrying the label which indicates enrichment.

Several approaches are in operation to relieve hunger and improve the nutritional status of all people in the United States. The school lunch program and the food enrichment program are striving toward such a goal. Advisors often hastily suggest that enrichment could supply all the needed nutrients; however, such a hasty enrichment could be dangerous when a major imbalance of nutrients is created. All professionals consider enrichment an effective technic if used with caution, care, and decisions based on research. "Elimination of hunger and malnutrition has moved to the forefront in national priorities," is a statement heard frequently these days. As an example, nutritionists estimate that as many as 40% of all females and many children may be suffering from iron deficiency anemia. In the fall of 1968, the Recommended Dietary Allowance (RDA) for iron was raised to a maximum of 18 mg, an amount which increased the RDA by 67%, which is to help offset the prevalence of iron deficiency. Naturally diet is considered as the solution. The protein foods supply about 40% of the iron in the

Table 2.1 Federal standards for enriched foods, 1969.

Standard for Enriched Macaroni Products

Required Ingredients per Pound of Flour

	Minimum	Maximum
Thiamine	4.0 milligrams	5.0 milligrams
Riboflavin	1.7 milligrams	2.2 milligrams
Niacin	27.0 milligrams	34.0 milligrams
Iron	13.0 milligrams	16.5 milligrams

Optional Ingredients

Calcium	500.0 milligrams	625.0 milligrams
Vitamin D	250 U.S.P. Units	1000 U.S.P. Units

Standard for Enriched Flour

Required Ingredients per Pound of Flour

	Minimum	Maximum
Thiamine	2.0 milligrams	2.5 milligrams
Riboflavin	1.2 milligrams	1.5 milligrams
Niacin	16.0 milligrams	20.0 milligrams
Iron	13.0 milligrams	16.5 milligrams

Optional Ingredients

Calcium	500.0 milligrams	625.0 milligrams
Vitamin D	250 U.S.P. Units	1000 U.S.P. Units

Standard for Enriched Self-Rising Flour

Required Ingredients per Pound of Flour

	Minimum	Maximum
Thiamine	2.0 milligrams	2.5 milligrams
Riboflavin	1.2 milligrams	1.5 milligrams
Niacin	16.0 milligrams	20.0 milligrams
Iron	13.0 milligrams	16.5 milligrams

Optional Ingredients

Calcium	500.0 milligrams	1500.0 milligrams
Vitamin D	250 U.S.P. Units	1000 U.S.P. Units

Standards for Enriched Rice

Required Ingredients per Pound

	Minimum	Maximum
Thiamine	2.0 milligrams	4.0 milligrams
Riboflavin	1.2 milligrams	2.4 milligrams
Niacin	16.0 milligrams	32.0 milligrams
Iron	13.0 milligrams	26.0 milligrams

From: Durum Wheat Institute (Dept. DWN F/69), 14 East Jackson Blvd., Chicago, Illinois 60604.

family dietary according to the USDA Survey (1965–1966) and cereal products supply an additional 30–40%. Obviously only cereal products lend themselves to iron fortification. Ironically, cereal products are not consumed in significant amounts by women and girls who need the iron supplementation.

One month before the start of the White House Conference on Food and Nutrition, on November 5, 1969, the milling and baking industries petitioned the Federal Food and Drug Administration for permission to triple the amount of biologically available iron specified in the Standards of Identity for enriched flours, bread, and bread-type rolls.

The iron petition reflected the concern and involvement of groups in business, agriculture, and government over mounting evidence of iron deficiency anemia, particularly among women of childbearing years and among children. At earlier meetings of millers, bakers, and wheat growers, with nutrition authorities, insufficient iron in diet came into sharp focus as the dietary problem of primary importance. The present standards for enriched flour require "not less than 13.0 mg and not more than 16.5 mg of iron." The petition asked that these levels be increased to read "not less than 50.0 mg and not more than 60 mg" per pound of enriched flour. The range for enriched bread, rolls, or buns is presently 8.0–12.5 mg. If the petition is accepted, these levels would be raised to 32.0–38.0 mg/lb per pound of bread. Present levels of enrichment from USDA Handbook No. 8 (1968) are given in Table 2.2 for comparison with unenriched and whole wheat values.

Table 2.2 Comparison of unenriched and enriched products with whole wheat ones.

	Thiamine mg/lb	Riboflavin mg/lb	Niacin mg/lb	Iron mg/lb
Bread:				
Unenriched with 1–2% nonfat dry milk	0.40	0.36	5.6	3.2
Enriched with 1–2% nonfat dry milk	1.13	0.77	10.4	10.9
Wh. Wheat with 2% nonfat dry milk	1.17	0.56	12.9	10.4
Flour–all purpose				
Unenriched	0.28	0.21	4.1	3.6
Enriched	2.00	1.20	16.0	13.0
Flour, whole wheat	2.49	0.54	19.7	15.0
80% extraction flour	1.16	0.33	9.3	5.9
Wheat germ	9.10	3.09	19.2	42.6

Data from USDA Handbook No. 8, Rev. 1963.

White Flour and Bread Enrichment was established by World War II Food Order No. 1 in May 1941 and required enrichment of all white flour and white bread.

School Lunch Program

The *National School Lunch Program* was created in 1947 with the aims of the School Lunch Act to:

1. give children a nutritionally adequate hot lunch at school,
2. serve as a means of distributing some farm surpluses,
3. train children and thereby families in good food habits.

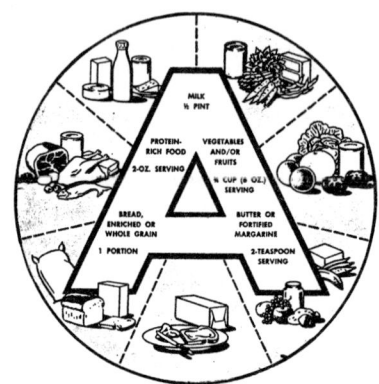

The requirements for *Type A School Lunch* were set so that the lunch supplied from one-third to one-half of the food needed daily by a child, which contains one-third to one-half of all nutrients required, not just bulk and calories. Adjustments need to be made in quantity for the younger child and especially for the high school teenager. A synopsis of the school lunch program is presented by Hill (1969) which includes the original National School Lunch Act. Public Law 396,

Fig. 2.5 Type A school lunch (data early in 1969 indicated that 1.7 million additional children to the 2.5 million regular participants were receiving the school lunch; "approximately 6 to 7 million children should be receiving nutritional assistance").

The Nation School Lunch Act, was approved June 4, 1946. The declaration of policy states:

> It is hereby declared to be the policy of Congress, as a measure of national security, to safeguard the health and well-being of the Nation's children, and to encourage the domestic consumption of nutritious agricultural commodities and other foods, by assisting the States, through grants-in-aid and other means, in providing an adequate supply of foods and other facilities for the establishment, maintenance, operation, and expansion of nonprofit school lunch programs.

Lunches served by school which comply with nutritional requirements specified are to be served to all children irrespective of ability to pay. The children are to receive lunches with anonymity for those who do not pay or pay only a portion of the cost. The nutritional quality which is

These quantities are for the 9–12-year-old boy or girl for each Type A School Lunch.

Milk — ½ pint as a beverage, more milk used in food preparation.	Supplies protein, calcium, vitamin A, thiamine, riboflavin, etc.
Protein food — 2 oz of lean meat, poultry, or fish; or meat substitutes; 2 oz cheese, one egg, ½ cup cooked dried beans or peas, 4 Tbsp. peanut butter.	Supplies protein, iron, B-vitamins and other nutrients.
Vegetables, fruit — ¾ c. consisting of 2 vegetables (1 green or yellow), 1 fruit.	Supplies vitamins A and C and others, iron, some calcium and good bulk.
Bread and cereal products — one slice of wholegrain or enriched bread; or a serving of other bread such as cornbread, biscuits, rolls, muffins, or bread made from wholegrain or enriched meal or flour, etc. Nonenriched products do not supply significant amounts of nutrients other than calories. Desserts should contain nutritious food, not just calories.	Wholegrain or enriched are good sources of calories since iron, thiamine, riboflavin, and other B vitamins are supplied. Calories without these nutrients are poor choices. Limit the pure calorie foods which are pure starch, pure fats, crackers, many bought cookies, cake flour, etc. Most commercial buns and doughnuts are nonenriched.
Butter — 2 tsp. of butter or fortified margarine.	Calories and vitamin A, other fats or shortenings have no vitamin A.

based on tested research, shall furnish one-third of the RDA for the age group involved. The school lunch is a food program. The pattern for the school lunch, even though originated in 1946, has remained the same in principle but has stressed greater recognition of individual food acceptance. Food must "look good and taste good" in order to promote participation and acceptability.

The present menu planning guide includes these recommendations:

1. a good source of vitamin A twice weekly,
2. a good source of vitamin C daily,
3. several sources of iron each day,
4. other foods to supply energy,
5. consideration of enhancing nutrient content by combinations of foods in a single serving,
6. since school lunches have been reported to be low in calories for children, well-chosen desserts are being developed such as ginger bread with apricot sauce.

The school lunch program provides lists of foods and recipes to help local managers meet these guides. Each food can be a "packet of nutrients" and thereby food groups are not specialists for specific nutrients but suppliers of multinutrient complexes. The fruit and vegetable group in Type A lunch presents the greatest range in nutrient value and is a good group to show the advantage of combinations of foods to make a more nutritious serving.

The food in the child is the only one to count; the child must learn to eat those foods he needs. The child who is taught to read is given a book; by the same token, "when a child is taught to eat, food is made available." Such experience for the child is not limited to the school lunch personnel who make the lunch available and encourage children to eat. The home and the classroom must help and cooperate with all aspects of the program. Children must learn "that good habits developed at home and in the lunch program are a good and enjoyable way to eat." Few school systems have developed a comprehensive program which incorporates the school lunch into the curriculum as a learning opportunity for children.

The principal of Woodlawn School in Portland, Oregon, Dr. Robert P. Selby, reported on efforts to incorporate the lunch as a nutrition education devise into the academic curriculum of schools. After several efforts were tried to achieve the best results, the outcomes were enumerated as follows:

1. More children ate a well-balanced nutritious lunch.
2. Plate waste was reduced.
3. Children ate a greater variety of food.
4. Children were less distracted by the noise of the previous lunch schedule.
5. Better harmonious relationships were developed resulting in reduced "arguments and disorders which formerly intruded into afternoon classes. ..."

In schools which have many children brought by buses for long distances, some breakfast feeding has been in practice for many years. More recently the breakfast program has been initiated into more school systems to meet dietary needs of children. It represents another step in the direction of public responsibility for child welfare.

Started April 1, 1970 amended regulations in the USDA school feeding program were to encourage private business expertise to design food service systems "airline style" to meet the dietary needs of school children. They were to propose ways which could be tried to bring the first adequate lunches to children in isolated rural areas or to inner city school children to eliminate poverty-related hunger and malnutrition. Over nine million children had no school lunch available in 1970, over 17 million are not eating school lunches; this leaves only about five million children participating. A staff of food inspectors and home economists in a USDA laboratory carefully test and analyze samples of fruits and vegetables selected for the National School Lunch Program to meet purchase specifications. The foods are tested for taste and appearance and to determine if they are suited for the purpose intended.

Who pays for the school lunch? Actually the cost is divided between several contributors; the children pay over half the cost, the state and local school program supply about 23% with the Federal donated food and cash subsidy contributing about 24%. The cost in 1969 was 59 cents per lunch per child, which is higher by 10 cents than in 1964.

The original purpose of the school lunch program was to improve the dietary practices of school children. This designates that the school lunch program financed 50% by tax money, must be more than a filling station: the school lunch must be part of the educational program of all school children. It represents a real-life situation for learning many meaningful experiences to assist the school child to develop socially and emotionally as well as physically through a balanced diet.

The future should expand the practice of enriching teaching with experiences involving food. Educators and nutritionists must continue to urge that the lunch experience be incorporated into the total school curriculum. This requires the understanding and cooperation of parents, school administrators, teachers, and the community.

Activities for Student Learning

1. You should view slides or look for pictures depicting how the development of technology has affected man's supply of available quality food. You may be interested in the early pioneers in the field of nutrition.

2. Analyze the current basic concepts of nutrition to determine which concepts you have acquired.

3. Suggest meaningful ways of teaching nutrition to children at different ages.

4. Students who want to learn nutrition should take advantage of such devices as this to keep up with new ideas and words:

Hot Tips:

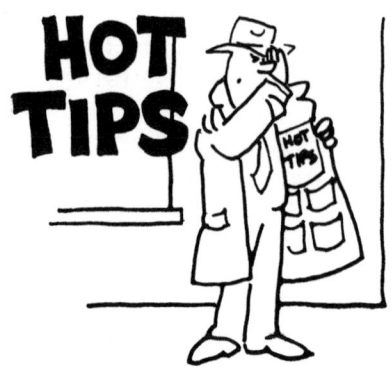

New Words:

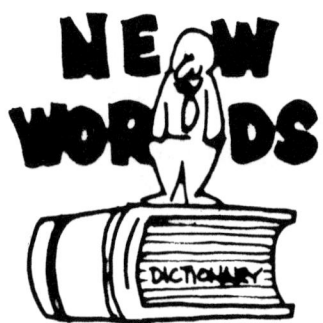

References and Suggested Readings

Basic Concepts in Nutrition Education, *Nutritional Program News.* Consumer and Food Economics Research Division, USDA, and the Interagency Committee Nutrition Education, Washington, D.C., 1967.

Berry, W. T. C. The problems of nutrition education, *Nutr. J. Dietet. Food Catering, and Child Nutr.,* **23**: 2, 10 (1969).

Carey, W. D. Panel Recommendations, *Nutr. Today,* **4**: 4, 16 (1969–70).

Enloe, C. H. Hitched to everything in the universe, *Nutr. Today,* **4**: 2, 2 (1970).

Eppright, E., *et al. Teaching Nutrition.* Ames, Iowa: Iowa State University Press, 1967.

The explorer and his food, *Nutr. Today.* **4**: 2, 3 (1969).

Farber, S. M., Wilson, N. L., and Wilson, R. H. *Food and Civilization: A Symposium.* Springfield, Ill.: Thomas, 1966.

Fry, D. H. Some thoughts on communication in nutrition teaching with particular reference to schools, *Nutr. J. Dietet., Food Catering and Child Nutr.,* **23**: 1, 10 (1969).

Hankin, J. Are teachers prepared to teach nutrition?, *J. Amer. Dietet. A.*, **25**: 8, 802 (1959).

Hill, M. M. Nutrition committees and nutrition education, *J. Nutr. Educ.*, **1**, 14 (1969).

Hill, M. M. The school lunch—a component of educational programs, *Nutrition Program News*. USDA, (November–December 1969).

Himsworth, H. What "nutrition" really means, *Nutr. Today*, **3**: 3, 18 (1968).

Jalso, S. B., Burns, M. M., and Rivers, J. M. Nutrition beliefs and practices, *J. Amer. Dietet. A.*, **47**, 263 (1965).

Lowenberg, M. E., *et al. Food and Man*. New York: Wiley, 1969.

Lyng, R. E. The government nutrition programs, the men in charge, *Nutr. Today*, **5**: 6, 16 (1970).

Lyng, R. E. The government's role in quality assurance, *Food Tech.*, **24**, 52 (1970).

Man's early knowledge of nutrition, *What's New in Home Eco.*, pp. 66–68 (1968).

Mayer, J. One year later, *J. Amer. Dietet. A.*, **58**, 300 (1971).

Maynard, L. A. Early days of nutrition research in the United States of America, *Nutr. Abtr. Rev.*, **32**, 345 (1962).

McCollum, E. V. *A History of Nutrition*. Boston: Houghton Mifflin, 1957.

Mertenes, M. W. Teaching therapeutic nutrition via independent study, *J. Amer. Dietet. A.*, **54**: 4, 302 (1969).

O'Hara, A. J. School feeding under an applied nutrition program, *Nutr. J. Dietet. Food Catering and Child Nutr.*, **22**: 1, 14 (1968).

Schubert, E. P. Nutrition Education: How much can or should our schools do?, *J. Nutr. Educ.*, **2**: 1, 9 (1970).

Sipple, J. L. The Nutrition Foundation—first twenty-five years, *Nutr. Rev.*, **24**, 353 (1966).

Symposium—landmarks of a half century of nutrition research, *J. Nutr.*, **91**, 1 (1967).

Thomas, L. From Eve to astronauts, *Nutr. Today*, **4**: 3, 5 (1969).

Tips for Teachers in Nutrition Education. Arizona State Department of Health, Maricopa County Health Department, Spring 1969.

Todhunter, E. N. Approaches to nutrition education, *J. Nutr. Educ.*, **1**: 1, 8 (1969).

Todhunter E. N. Development of knowledge in nutrition, *J. Amer. Dietet. A.*, **44**, 100 (1964).

USDA, Food consumptions of households in the United States, Spring 1965, Report No. 1., U.S. Govt. Ptg. Office, ARS-34, 1968.

White House Conference on Food, Nutrition, and Health, Dec. 2–4, 1969, Final Report, 1970, Supt. Doc., Washington, D.C., 1970.

INVENTORY OF KNOWLEDGE

Part I Matching

From the list on the right *select* the best answer for the description given on the left; place your answer in the space that is provided.

A. Man's concern for food has changed through the ages and is reflected in the technological developments.

_____ 1. Initiated the use of horsepower to replace manpower

_____ 2. Learned to make weapons from stones

(a) The Forager
(b) The Hunter
(c) The Agrarian

_____ 3. Began to migrate and search for "more"
and "different" food

_____ 4. Concerned about how to help those less
fortunate than himself

_____ 5. Referred to as a peasant, a peon

_____ 6. Instigated the creation of an abundance of food and fiber

_____ 7. Concerned about mass populations

_____ 8. Implemented the idea of land-grant colleges

(d) The Industrialist
(e) The Scientific
(f) The Humanitarian

B. Nutrition is a relative "newcomer" to the field of science; however, a vast
number of people have contributed to the current knowledge of nutrition. If
these facts are not familiar to you look them up in a reference book.

_____ 9. Named the yellow pigment found in corn

_____10. Identified the amino acid, methionine

_____11. Coined the word vitamine

_____12. Published the first U.S. bulletin on the
composition of foods

_____13. Developed the concept of dietary standards,
predecessor to the NRC's RDA

_____14. Fed cattle on limited ratios "to locate a
nutrient due to its absence"

_____15. Established the oath used in medicine and also related body heat
production to growth, age, and activity

_____16. In 1969 directed the largest nutrition conference ever held

(a) Rose
(b) McCollum
(c) Hippocrates
(d) Funk
(e) Mayer
(f) Atwater
(g) Sherman

Part II   Multiple Choice

Circle the letter of the best choice for completion of each statement:

17. Examples of legislative regulations which have improved the health of United
States citizens include the:
    (a) establishment of land-grant colleges
    (b) creation of the HEW Department
    (c) passage of the Smith-Hughes Act
    (d) planning of White House Conferences on nutrition and related areas
    (e) all of the above

18. The national concern about nutrition in the United States has been publicized by:
    (a) conferences which consider the nutritional status of all the people
    (b) a government that is interested in the well-being of its citizens
    (c) the realization that malnutrition does exist within this country
    (d) the sharing of concern by industry, the health professions, the mass media, churches, etc.
    (e) all of the above

19. When developing the Four Basic Concepts in Nutrition, the ICNE defined concepts as:
    (a) meanings that direct a person's responses and his decisions to problems
    (b) springboards for program planning for enrichment
    (c) the foods that you like and how to prepare them
    (d) a fad in educational jargon
    (e) the bases for formulating a testing program

20. Enrichment laws adopted by certain states in the United States promise that:
    (a) thiamine, riboflavin, niacin, and iron have been added to foods
    (b) all family or all purpose flour and white bread are enriched
    (c) sanitary food facilities are provided for the customer
    (d) periodic health examinations are conducted for food service employees
    (e) vitamin content of food is regulated by government

21. Of major concern to nutrition authorities is the deficiency of iron in the diet of some *women* and *children*. The remedy for this problem that has been suggested is to:
    (a) add iron to the list of nutrients required by the enrichment law
    (b) raise the RDA for iron to a minimum of 15 mg for adult males
    (c) fortify meats and meat products with iron
    (d) increase the levels of iron already required by the enrichment law
    (e) increase the daily food intake

22. The purposes of the National School Lunch Program include:
    (a) furnishing more than one-half of the child's nutritional needs
    (b) distributing some of the farm surplus products
    (c) serving a nutritionally adequate hot lunch
    (d) training children to develop good food habits
    (e) answers (b), (c), and (d)

23. The National School Type A Lunch must include certain types of foods. Which of the following food groups must be included to meet the criteria for this type of lunch?
    (a) $\frac{1}{2}$ pint of milk, 2 oz meat, serving of vegetable and bread
    (b) 8 oz of milk, a calcium rich food source. 4 Tbsp. peanut butter
    (c) iced tea, an iron rich food source, 2 oz cheese
    (d) $\frac{1}{2}$ pint of chocolate milk, a calcium rich food source. 3 oz meat
    (e) 4 oz of whole milk, an iron rich food source, 2 oz meat.

3

Growth and Development as Indicators of Nutritional Status

How Do Growth and Development reflect the Nutritional Status Achieved by an Individual?

Each person is the total of his life's nutrition. Deficits of certain nutrients at specific times affect developmental success within the genetic potential of a person, for example, the specific developmental sequence of tooth formation. The tooth structures for both deciduous and permanent teeth are formed during a short period of the life-span beginning prenatally, continuing during childhood, and reaching completion in adolescence. The required nutrient balance is most crucial during this period for the teeth to achieve the genetic potential of the individual. Thus a close alliance between nutrient need and physical development needs to be understood and stressed in nutrition education.

Much confusion has been evident in an effort to balance the supply of dietary nutrients with signs of nutritional status. Nutritional aberrations do not give prompt outward signs of malfunction so that they often are not recognized even by skilled medical diagnosticians. Constantly the technics of identification of subclinical symptoms are being refined to help to assure diagnosis and early treatment. In the past, too often the practice has been either to give massive dosage of some nutrient for no specific symptom or to disregard the need for therapy of any kind.

DEVELOPMENTAL PROGRESS OF MAN

Objectives

1. To recall that growth and maturation involve orderly, systematic increments of increased body size and function terminating in the stature of the adult.
2. To be aware that failure in any stage of the growth process may have a permanent-irreversible effect on the stature and performance of the individual as an adult.
3. To identify signs of health and of malnutrition during growth and development in children.
4. To compare the multiple parameters which influence an individual's optimum growth: the ecology of nutritional status.

Growth Patterns

Growth is an orderly sequence of events which produces an adult in a specified time. Growth is not only an increase in size and total mass but also maturation of functional aspects of development. The 1970s will bring clarification of the relationship of growth and maturation of the brain which represents probably the first tissue complex to reach maturity in the body. Thus the skull shows the most development prior to birth and the least growth afterwards in attaining adult size as can be noted in Fig. 3.1 and Fig. 3.2. Obviously skull growth is required for brain growth. Medical histories have shown retarded skull development to have caused damaged brain function. From birth to adulthood, the head enlarges twice the birth size, the trunk three times, the arm four times, and the legs five times the length. A person's adult height can be

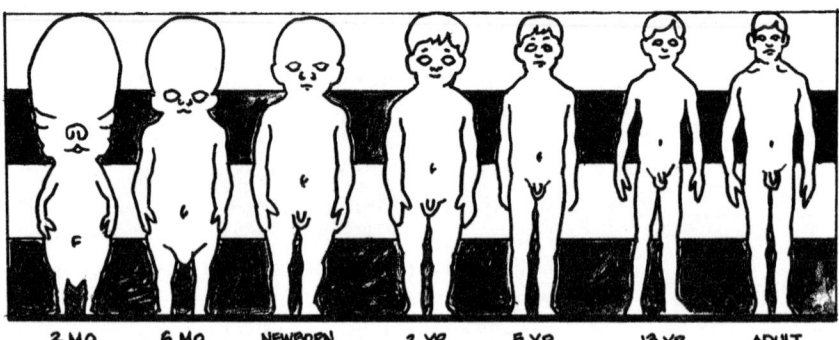

| 2 MO | 6 MO | NEWBORN | 2 YR | 5 YR | 13 YR | ADULT |

Fig. 3.1 Rates of physical enlargement with age.

predicted by multiplying by two the height at age $2\frac{1}{2}$–3 years. In Fig. 3.1 the head makes up half of the length of the two-month-old embryo where it represents less than one-eighth of the adult. Other dimensions can be compared. The shaded areas behind the adult figure are the size of that structure in the newborn in Fig. 3.2.

Growth and differentiation of structure are always in an anterior-posterior direction; the head forms first, the posterior parts follow. The arms and hands develop earlier and faster than do the legs and feet. Changes in bone development occur until an individual is about 20 years old when the skeleton is considered mature.

Since little is known about maturation patterns of soft tissues, the skeleton is commonly used as an indication of growth. Linear growth is used to measure the total progress the body is making toward maturity and is considered a reliable index. Relatively little analysis is made of the

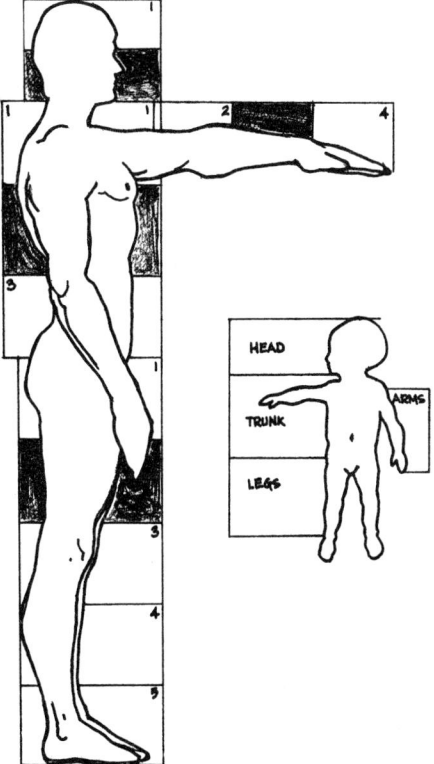

Fig. 3.2 Proportionate difference between newborn and adult.

proportionate growth of all the parts, namely, trunk length or sitting height in contrast to total height, of leg and arm length related to trunk length. Examples of short or long legged individuals are common and often the focus of jokes such as "Tell Joe to stand up," or "Have Jim get down off the chair."

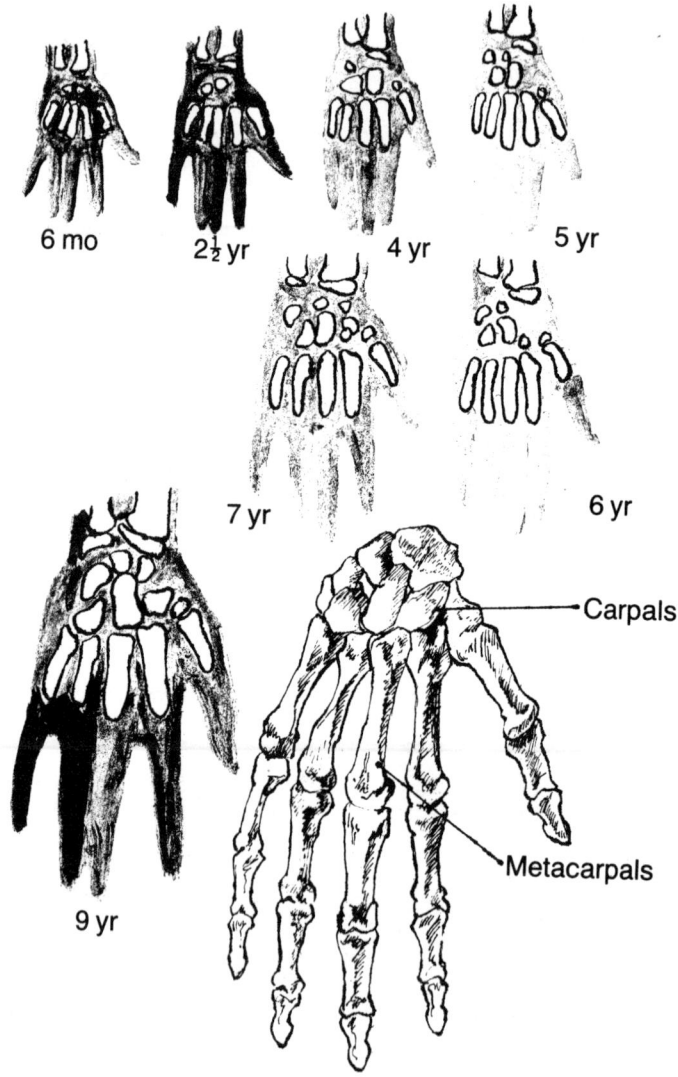

Fig. 3.3   The stages of maturation.

Medical and human developmental scientists judge skeletal maturation by identification of carpals as shown in Fig. 3.3. Carpal bone development differs for boys and girls. The fifth carpal bone in the wrist
develops in the average girl at four years, but in the average boy at five
years. No bony carpals are present at birth; by puberty all eight small
bones are formed. Maturation occurs independently of mineralization of
bone; the presence of ossification centers does not assure adequate bone
structure and explains the development of rickets which may occur in an
apparently average growth pattern.

Physical performance in infants is dependent on growth and skeletal
development. The closure of the fontanel indicates skeletal maturation
as well as mineralization. Normally this "anterior soft spot" in an infant's
head closes as age increases. One can visualize that normal performance
of infants is dependent on skeletal growth and consequently on a sufficient nutrient supply at all times during this period of rapid body change.
Physical performance dependent on growth and skeletal development is
used as an indicator of maturation.

Growth and Nutrition of the Young Child

Genetics is the architect but nutrition is the builder; dietetics is the
provision of food with proper nutrient content and acceptable to the
people involved. Some people attain their genetic potential; many do
not. Average birth weight of a child is influenced by the nutrition of the
mother even prior to conception. Sufficient supply of nutrients, both in
amount and ratio to each other, in the maternal blood, and consequently
in placental blood, is crucial to growth and development throughout
prenatal life. The proportionate size of embryonic and fetal growth
prior to the sixth month of pregnancy requires little additional nutrient
intake to that needed by the mother
for her normal life; however, increased amounts of nutrients are
highly necessary for the last trimester. Calories intake needs to
meet only energy expenditure in
order that the gain in weight will
be the result of growth of tissues
involved in pregnancy and not from
increase in adipose tissues.

Growth in the first year of life
is comparatively uniform among

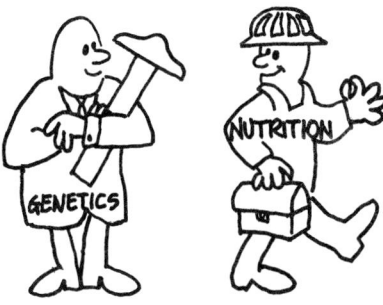

Fig. 3.4 Genetics is the architect but
nutrition is the builder.

people because infants are relatively well fed on a milk diet whether human beings, cows milk, or formula diets. Limited amounts of iron and ascorbic acid in milk require these milk diets to be supplemented after a few weeks. Foods fed to infants and young children need to educate them in food acceptance and to train them in sound food habits while at the same time supplying nutrients sufficient for their potential growth.

The Ecology of Human Nutrition

Nutrition is the product of many parameters affecting the life of an individual, of a family, or of an ethnic group. One has difficulty in visualizing what life would be if parents had lived elsewhere – in the tropics, in the arctic, in an undeveloped nation, in an isolated region, or in poverty at the perimeter of a vast city. Have you expressed appreciation for the environmental ecology of your origin which permitted you to be a student? To consider the total ecology of nutritional status, first consider the major parameters which determine whether a given family or person is well fed. Naturally, *food is fundamental*: the availability of an assortment of food which will supply needed nutrients, that is of safe quality and in the amount required by each age group. This food supply *depends on individual people* who also must know to *establish allied health services* which are oriented to the human being. These three areas are the ABC's of the nutritional status of a person. Furthermore, to support such a status requires multiple areas of concern culminating in a "good government" which is a servant and tool of the people involved. Obviously, good government is dependent on the same institutions which it fosters. These concepts are presented in Table 3.1. The fact is often overlooked that an individual is not in control of his destiny, not an island unto himself, but is partially the victim of other factors of environment. These influences actually start prior to conception and continue during both prenatal and postnatal life. A person is the product of his parents and their genetic and cultural heritage in addition to their social values and educational achievement. The food supply depends on the geographic resources, man's utilization of natural assets and on the government. Sanitation, health services, and educational level of citizens are all related to government, whether autocratic and selfish or democratic and public spirited.

The same type of analogy can be made for the ecology of malnutrition as given in Table 3.2. The fact that people are not all in the same state of malnutrition depends on the multiple facets of parentage, the geographic location, and the type of government sponsored by the society.

Table 3.1   The ecology of human nutrition. (The ABC's of Nutritional Status are Supported by Social Values, Education, the Community, Business, and Good Government.)

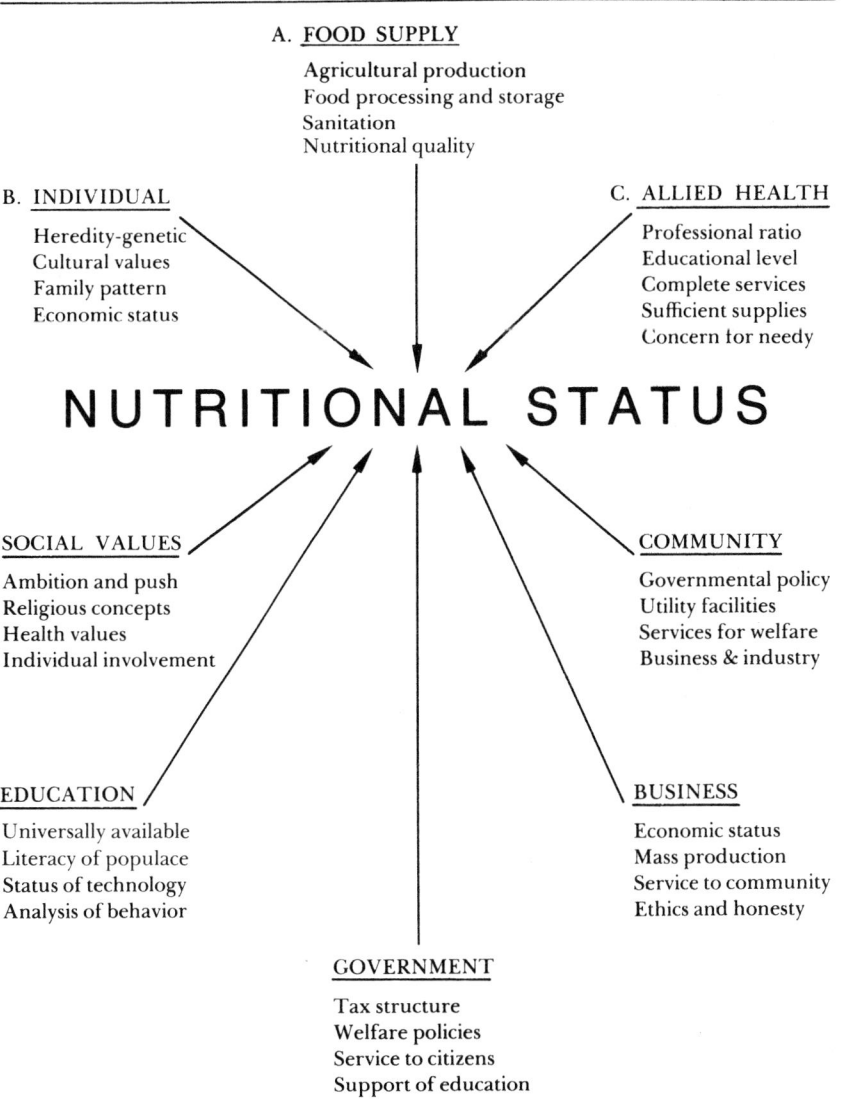

A. FOOD SUPPLY

Agricultural production
Food processing and storage
Sanitation
Nutritional quality

B. INDIVIDUAL

Heredity-genetic
Cultural values
Family pattern
Economic status

C. ALLIED HEALTH

Professional ratio
Educational level
Complete services
Sufficient supplies
Concern for needy

NUTRITIONAL STATUS

SOCIAL VALUES

Ambition and push
Religious concepts
Health values
Individual involvement

COMMUNITY

Governmental policy
Utility facilities
Services for welfare
Business & industry

EDUCATION

Universally available
Literacy of populace
Status of technology
Analysis of behavior

BUSINESS

Economic status
Mass production
Service to community
Ethics and honesty

GOVERNMENT

Tax structure
Welfare policies
Service to citizens
Support of education

Table 3.2   Ecology of malnutrition.

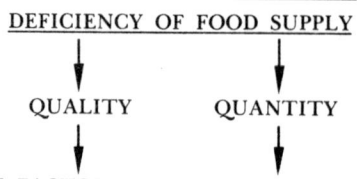

DEFICIENCY OF FOOD SUPPLY

QUALITY   QUANTITY

MULTIPLE FACTORS WHICH AFFECT FOOD SUPPLY
Geography and natural resources
Climatic and environmental limitations
Governmental policies toward agriculture
Agricultural development and production
Scientific technological development
Industrial food processing (preservation)
Customs and culture
Safety of food in storage and service

ECONOMICS

Limited natural resources
Lack of industry
Unemployment
Limited income
Many dependents

DISEASES

Parasites
Infections; fevers
Ignorance in treatment:
    excess use of purgatives
    witchcraft
    medical quackery

MALNUTRITION

GOVERNMENT

Lack of concern for majority
Few wealthy, many poor people
Limited services – health, roads
    education, welfare, sanitation

MEDICAL SERVICES

Limited trained personnel
Incompetent workers
Limited supplies & facilities
Primitive concepts

COMMUNITY

Generally unsanitary environment
Limited educational opportunity
Familial clannishness
Lack of awareness of needs
Limited resources

EDUCATION

General illiteracy
Limited education in all areas
Limited communication
    between areas or the world

PSYCHOLOGICAL FACTORS
Lack of change
Attachment to the past
Inexperience in creativity
Fears and superstitions
Lack of group activity

Characteristics of a Person with the Malnutrition Syndrome

People whose food supply has been deficient because of one or more of the multiple factors listed in Table 3.2 will exhibit certain distinctive traits which are summarized as follows:

1. highly abnormal height-weight ratios — emaciation or obesity;
2. pallor — low hemoglobin levels and/or low erythrocyte count;
3. weary, worried facial expression — hollow cheeks, circles around eyes, apathetic and depressed rejection;
4. postural slump — drooping shoulders, winged back, hollow chest, malalignment of skeleton and protruding stomach;
5. neglect and indifference about personal appearance and habits of cleanliness — loss of pride, self-esteem, and confidence;
6. slow indecisive movements — muscular weakness, lack of neuro-muscular coordination, accident-prone, and fatigued;
7. mental dullness and lack of alert response — deficient quality of blood supply to brain increases inaccurate responses, errors and accidents;
8. lack of appetite — feeling of fullness and rejection of a variety of food;
9. certain symptoms evident in the skin — chronic sore mouth and tongue, glossitis, prickling burning of skin, stomatitis, cheilosis, and general dermatitis;
10. red swollen easily bleeding sore gums;
11. lacrimation with burning, itching, and a discharge accumulation on eyelid, abnormal light tolerance (photophobia), and night blindness;
12. muscle tenderness, cramps, and pains especially in the joints — poor muscle tone and change in reflexes;
13. enlargement of joints accompanied by pain and edema — deformed shape of bones and alignment of skeleton;
14. general nervousness and irritability;
15. chronic diarrhea and sudden death.

A study of the ecological aspects of either nutritional status or of malnutrition emphasizes the fact that malnutrition is not a single concept but a syndrome, a group of symptoms that occur together to characterize a disease. The trend has been to treat one symptom of malnutrition alone, the treatment depending on the "specialist's" viewpoint. To give a child a lunch at school does not eradicate his or his family's problem of malnutrition because the value of the lunch depends on whether he eats it and whether he learns, or is able, to choose meals for himself at home and elsewhere which are as nutritionally well balanced. The lunch alone is only a temporary treatment. Much of the "do-good" of welfare has not produced any change in behavior but has only pacified the recipient.

Obviously, many factors are involved in promoting and maintaining the health of the individuals in any country. Adult females seem to withstand privation of food supplies better than men and often exhibit highly excessive fat deposits. The younger the child the lower will be his survival if food supplies are insufficient to meet his physiological needs. Obviously, unsanitary conditions, diseases, and lack of protection from adverse weather increase the damage caused by limited amount and variety of food.

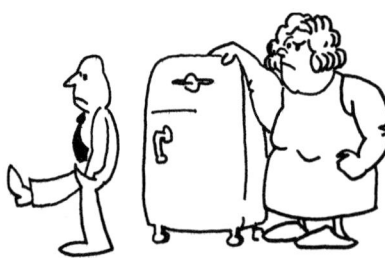

Fig. 3.5 Adult females can withstand starvation better than males.

Probably the outstanding example of nations with a similar ecology of nutritional status combining their efforts to face the multiple aspects of adequate nutrition, is the group which organized the Institute of Nutrition of Central America and Panama (INCAP) with its headquarters at Guatemala City, Guatemala. This organization published a series of diagrams, one to stress the interrelationships of nutritionists and other specialists concerned about nutrition; another to emphasize the three faceted cycle of those sciences responsible for food production, those of socioeconomic marketing and consumer acceptance of food and those of the allied health fields. The last schema indicated that over 20 areas are involved and that no one person can comprehend or participate in all areas of involvement. The solution to the dilemma is the team approach in which specialists from each unique area cooperate.

Activities for Student Learning

1. You should read sections from textbooks describing growth patterns and hypothesize as to retardation that can result from certain nutrient deficiencies or from a general lack of sufficient food.
2. Work with a partner to compare body sizes of different groups in the world populations, such as Japanese, Swedish, Indian, African, and "United Statesans." How could this be explained in relation to nutrition?

3. You need to use the chart, *Ecology of Human Nutrition* to explain *your* nutritional status; explain that of another ethnic group.
4. You need to be able to relate characteristics of people with different food consumption to students who have dietary habits resulting from poor food choices or fad diets.
5. You might want to view the filmstrip — "Your Food Chance or Choice," prepared by the National Dairy Council, Chicago. Illinois.

ASSESSMENT OF BODY SIZE

Objectives

1. To relate the concept of "average weight" of a body for a given height, build, age, and sex.
2. To identify that the genetic potential for human size can be altered by inadequate nutrition during growth.
3. To develop skill in the assessment of body size as related to age, body composition, frame size, daily variability, and sex.

Height-Weight-Age Ratios

Height-weight-age ratios have been the traditional device by which to judge growth and physical well-being. The discrepancies encountered have caused a rather negative attitude by many researchers toward the reliability of these ratios. For more than 50 years, these ratios have been merely averages of measurements on people of undetermined health. These averages are not ideal for everyone but are simply midpoints between maxima and minima of measurements on people and no data are available to ascertain if this midpoint is a measurement of a period of optimum health. Average height-weight-age tables, therefore, are being modified in order to allow for differences in body build, although a method of determining build has not been put into general use. Only a few people in the allied medical field allow for some specified deviation from the average weight to be considered "normal"

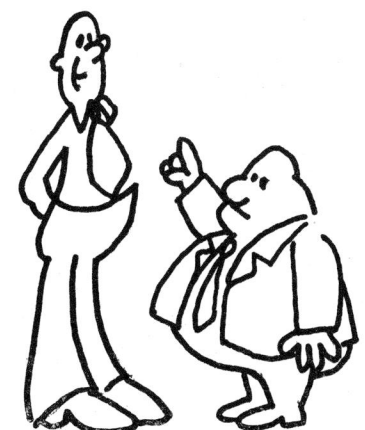

Fig. 3.6 Average size is not ideal for anyone.

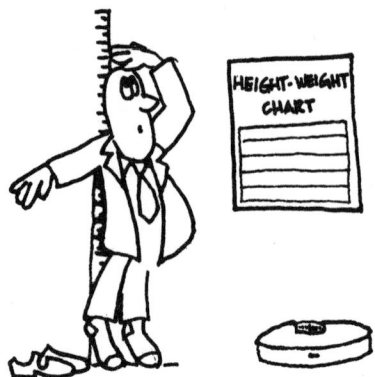

Fig. 3.7   All too often the correct weight is considered a single absolute value.

or desirable. All too often correct weight is considered a single absolute value.

The height-weight-age ratio alone is a very poor criterion by which to judge growth or well-being. Suggested modifications by definition of body build, range of normalcy, and desirable weight greatly add to its validity. Research is in progress to develop other measurements.

The growth in height of the "reference person" and the proportional weight as established by the NRC's RDA in 1968 is diagrammed in Fig. 3.8.

Definitions of Body Size

Since various terminology is used in describing the size of the human body, definitions for body size need to be understood.

For Children

1. Average weight for a child is the predicted weight for a given height and sex as published by the Metropolitan Life Insurance Company. This average is sometimes designated as "normal" recommended weight.

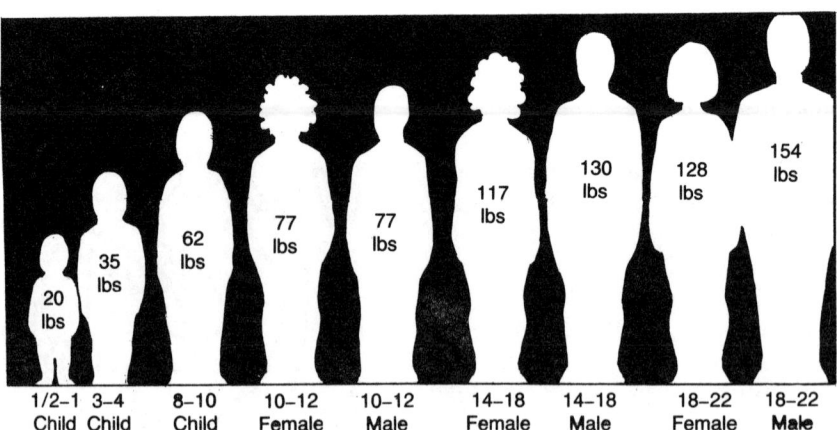

Fig. 3.8   Growth in height of the "Reference Man" at different ages.

2. Zones are given in Taylor and Pye (1966) based on data originally published by Joint Committee on Health Problems in Education of NEA and AMA.
3. Desirable weight for children is that which supports regular increments of growth and a moderate layer of subcutaneous fat.

For Adults

1. Average weight for an adult is determined by the same method as used for the child.
2. A range of weight has been specified as acceptable for adults as + or −10% of the average weight.
3. Desirable or ideal weight for adults is the normal weight at age 22 if the individual is healthy at that time.
4. Overweight is any weight more than 10% and up to 20% above average weight.
5. Obesity is 20% or more above average weight.

Zones of normalcy of weight during the life-cycle can be illustrated as in Fig. 3.9.

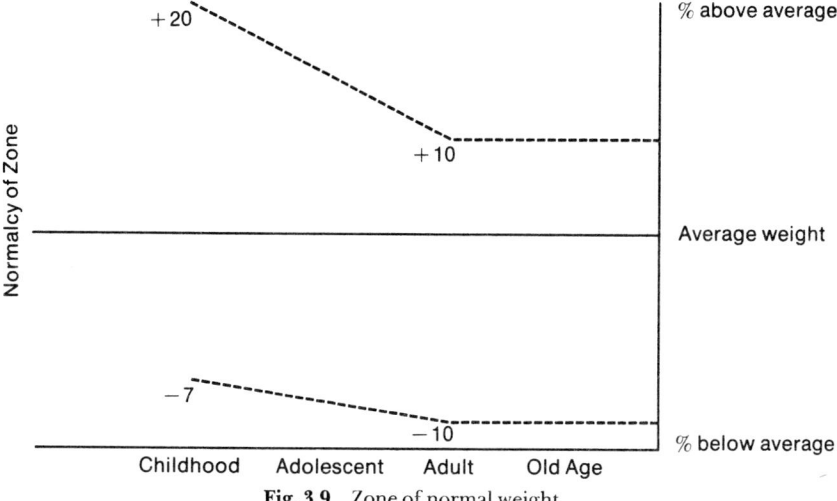

Fig. 3.9 Zone of normal weight.

Maintenance of desirable weight can be achieved when the calorie requirement for each adult is calculated from a formula based on *desired weight* (W) which is the average weight of the person at age 22 considering his weight, frame size, and sex (1968 revision of NRC's Recommended Dietary Allowances).

$$\text{Calories for men} = 0.95\,(815 + 36.6\,W)$$
$$\text{Calories for women} = 0.95\,(580 + 31.1\,W)$$

Frame Size Estimation

To date, no simple formula has been designated by which to calculate frame size. Morton (1964) quoted Louis Hippe (Warner Bros.); "The wrist varies with one's bones, and on the weight and size of these depends the correct measurement of each person." The following data are given by permission of John Wiley & Sons, Inc.:

Louis Hippe's "Rule of the Wrist"

Chest measures $5\frac{1}{2}$ times the wrist
Waist measures 4 times the wrist
Hips measures 6 times the wrist
Thigh measures $3\frac{1}{2}$ times the wrist
Calf measures $2\frac{1}{2}$ times the wrist
Ankle measures $1\frac{1}{4}$ times the wrist

Circumference of wrist in inches

Height	Small-Boned	Medium-Boned	Large-Boned
Under 5'3"	Less than $5\frac{1}{2}"$	$5\frac{1}{2}$ to $5\frac{3}{4}"$	Over $5\frac{3}{4}"$
5'4"	Less than 6"	6 to $6\frac{1}{4}"$	Over $6\frac{1}{4}"$
Over 5'4"	Less than $6\frac{1}{4}"$	$6\frac{1}{4}$ to $6\frac{1}{2}"$	Over $6\frac{1}{2}"$

Weight adjustment for bone size:

Medium-boned persons; start with 5 foot height and 110 pound weight, add 5 pounds for each additional inch of height.

Small-boned persons; deduct 10 pounds from the weight of medium-boned persons of the same height.

Large-boned persons; add 10 pounds to the weight of a medium-boned person of the same height.

From research by Lamb, Kassouny, and Brittin reported in *Proceedings of 7th International Nutrition Congress*, 1966, the following formula for frame size index was presented:

FSI (Frame size index) $= 0.262803\,(X1) + 12.370797\,(X2) + 4.342704\,(X3)$

Where X1 = weight in kg
X2 = wrist circumference in cm
X3 = chest diameter in cm minus scapular skinfold

An index below 260.97 would be small frame;
from 260.97 to 286.25 would be medium frame;
above 286.25 would be large frame.

This formula was based on the minimum predictors for frame size and the results correlated closely with other formulas based on a larger number of body measurements.

Other means of determining "normalcy" of size are suggested almost daily, such as the suggestion that the difference in height and waistline measured in inches should be 36; if more than 38 then leanness is indicated and if 33 or less then obesity. Measurement for height should be without shoes for women; measurement for waist without girdle and during exhalation.

Body Composition

Body composition is a reliable reflection of calorie balance, growth, musculature, health, and vigor; a criterion of total well-being for both children and adults. One needs to be alert to new findings in interpretation of data on body composition and physical measurements for use in assessment of nutritional status and health.

The body is composed of bone, muscle, water, and adipose deposits in decreasing order of density (weight per unit volume). For a 65 kg man, 25 years old, the average composition of this body is as follows:

Total Body Weight	
Water	61%
Protein	17%
Fat	14%
Minerals	7%
Carbohydrates	1%

The average 25-year-old woman has a higher ratio of fat in the body, about 25% is reported. Furthermore, Davidson and Passmore report in *Human Nutrition and Dietetics* that in an obese person, the fat stores can represent up to 70% of the total body weight. The percentage of fat in individuals in their fifties has been shown to be twice that at age 25.

Adipose tissue is the deposit of fat (triglycerides) into specialized cells (the number is determined by genetic inheritance). This tissue is either visceral or subcutaneous fat; the latter is the offender in development of obesity. The measurement of subcutaneous fat in selected areas of the body is becoming of paramount value in identifying the extent of obesity at any age, namely, the skinfold test, popularly termed the "pinch test." Further information about skinfold measurements is supplied by the references listed at the end of this chapter.

Losing Pounds — How Many and How Fast: Approximately 3500 calories are in each stored pound of fat. Thus to lose one pound a week, one should consume 500 fewer calories each day than expended or the reverse procedure to gain weight. Figure it this way . . .

> 150 pounds desired weight
> ×15 calories per pound for moderate activity/day
> 2250 calories needed to maintain desired weight
> −500 calories daily deficit to lose one pound per week
> 1750 maximum daily calories to be eaten to lose one pound per week

If two pounds each week are to be lost, the calculation would simply be:

> 150 pounds desired weight
> ×15 calories per pound for moderate activity/day
> 2250 calories need to maintain desired weight
> −1000 calories daily deficit
> 1250 maximum daily calories to be eaten to lose two pounds per week

To try to lose more than two pounds per week is usually unwise because a rapid weight loss may leave a person tired, grumpy, and vulnerable to illness. If a person is more than 10 pounds overweight, the family doctor should be consulted before launching any do-it-yourself reducing diet. Many people who are overweight or obese have unsuspected illnesses and to diet would be foolhardy and may complicate an already serious condition by depriving the body of the nutrition it needs.

Activities for Student Learning

1. Work with a partner to measure, record, and evaluate each student's analyses of body size. Each student should determine and record these measurements and analyses using the spaces provided on page 55.
   (a) weight in indoor clothing without shoes
   (b) height without shoes
   (c) skinfolds as indicators of subcutaneous fat
   (d) wrist circumference as indicator of frame size
   (e) predicted body weight
2. View slides or other visual aids showing a variety of body compositions and structures.
3. Read from the references list.
4. Interpret the maintenance or change in your body conformation that would be desirable and prepare a brief, well constructed summation. Complete the measurements and calculations to show your deviations from recommended body size and composition.

1. Name _____ .

2. Age _____ .

3. Weight _____ pounds _____ kg.

4. Height _____ inches _____ cm.

5. Skinfold measurements:

   (a) *For scapular measurement* on the back of a person locate the tip of the right scapula.

   For arm measurement locate a midpoint between the acromial tip of the scapula and the tip of the elbow over the triceps muscle, with the arm flexed at 90 degrees.

   (b) Lift the skinfold parallel to the length of the body and apply caliper one inch from edge to fold.

   (c) Read dial of caliper in mm thickness of the fold.

   Scapular skin fold _____ mm Triceps skinfold _____ mm.

6. Bone measurements:

   (a) Wrist circumference: measure with a steel tape preferable between hand and tip of ulna.

   Wrist circumference _____ in. _____ cm.

   (b) Estimation of frame size:

   Wrist circumference _____ Frame size index (FSI) _____ .

7. Determine the predicted or recommended body weight based on height, age, frame size, and sex as indicated.

   Predicted weight _____ lb   Actual weight _____ lb.

   Difference Plus _____ lb _____ %   or   Minus _____ lb _____ %.

References and Suggested Readings

Brozek, J. *Human Body Composition.* New York: Pergamon, 1965.

Brozek, J., Grande, F., Anderson, J. T., and Keys, A. *Densitometric Analysis of Body Composition: Revision of Some Quantitative Assumptions.* Ann. New York Acad. Sci., **110**: 113 (1963).

Davidson, L. S. P., and Passmore, R. *Human Nutrition and Dietetics.* Baltimore: Williams & Wilkins, 1966.

Dwyer, J. T., Feldman, J. J., Seltzer, C. C., and Mayer, J. Adolescent attitudes toward weight and appearance, *J. Nutr. Educ.*, **1**: 2, 14 (1969).

The effect of nutrition on body composition, *Dairy Council Digest*, **37**: 1 (1966).

Dayton, D. H. Early nutrition and human development, *Children*, **16**: 210 (1969).

Experimental epidemiology: Nutrition and infection, *Nutr. Rev.*, **27**: 306 (1969).

Hashim, S. A., and Van Itallie, T. B. Clinical and physiological aspects of obesity, *J. Am. Dietet. A.*, **46**: 15 (1965).

Hutson, E. M., Cohen, N. L., Kunkel, N. D., Steinkamp, R. C., Rourke, M. H., and Walch, H. E. Measures of body fat and related factors in normal adults, *J. Am. Dietet. A.*, **47**: 179 (1965).

Lamb, Mina W., Kassouny, M., and Brittin, H. Frame size as a determinant in judging adequacy of weight. Proceedings of 7th International Nutr. Congress, Vol. 4, Hamburg, Germany, 1966.

Martin, P. C., and Vincent, E. L. *Human Development*. New York: Ronald Press, 1960.

Mayer, J. The physiological basis of obesity and leanness, Part II, *Nutr. Abstr. Rev.*, **25**: 871 (1955).

Mayer, Jean. Physical activity and anthropometric measurements of obese adolescents, *Fed. Proc.*, **25**: 11 (1966).

Morton, A. *The Arts of Costume and Personal Appearance*, 3rd ed. New York: Wiley, 1964.

Overweight: It's prevention and significance. A series of articles reprinted from *Statistical Bulletin*. Metropolitan Life Insurance Company, 1960.

Seltzer, C. C., Goldman, R. F., and Mayer, J. The triceps skinfold as a predictive measure of body density and body fat in obese adolescent girls, *Pediatrics*, **36**: 2, 212 (1965).

Seltzer, C. C., and Mayer, J. A simple criterion of obesity, *Post-grad. Med.*, **38**: 101, 1965.

Skerli, B., Brozek, J., and Junt, E. E., Jr. Subcutaneous fat and age changes in body form in women, *Amer. J. Phys. Anthro.*, (N.S.) **11**, 577 (1953).

Steinkamp, R. C. Measured body fat, dietary practices and physical activity in healthy adults, *Food and Nutr. News*, National Livestock and Meat Board, **36**: 4 (January 1965).

Tanner, J. M. *Human Growth*. New York: Pergamon, 1969.

Task Force Action Statement. *Nutr. Today*, **4**: 4, 2 (1970).

Taylor, C. M., and Pye, V. *Foundations of Nutrition*. New York: Wiley, 1966.

Wart, B., Blair, R., and Roberts, L. J. Energy intake of well-nourished children and adolescents, *Amer. J. Clin. Nutr.*, **22**: 1383 (1969).

Weight Control Source Book. Chicago: National Dairy Council, 1967.

Zones of normalcy, Joint Committee on Health Problems in Education of NEA and AMA, *Amer. J. Pub. Health*, **39**, 878 (1949).

INVENTORY OF KNOWLEDGE

Part I

Complete the following statements by filling in the blanks with the appropriate terms:

1. Food makes a difference since each person is the total of his life's _____.

2. Growth is an orderly sequence of events, probably the first tissue complex to reach maturity in the body is the _____ tissue. The one most developed prior to birth and the least afterwards in order to attain adult size is _____.

3. Growth and differentiation of human structure are always in an _____ – _____ direction. The structural system that may be used as an indication of growth is the _____ . A more critical determination of maturity is possible by identifying the development of the _____ _____ in the _____ .

4. The architect is the _____ , but _____ is the builder; _____ is the provision of acceptable food with the proper nutrient content.

5. Growth of infants is comparatively uniform and regular because of a common diet consisting mainly of milk; however, supplements required early in life are _____ and _____ _____ .

6. Nutritional status is the product of many parameters; principal determinants are: _____ that is available to people, the _____ of the person, especially that of the mother, and freedom from _____ to reduce diarrhea.

Part II

The "ABC's of Nutritional Status" are affected by other parameters; match the following by choosing *one* or *more terms* from those on the right to match each description:

	Description	*Term*
_____	7. quality of food depends on honesty and integrity	(a) Social values
_____	8. "keep up with the Jones'es"	(b) Education
_____	9. support of education depends on tax structure	(c) Community
_____	10. initiation of welfare plans and programs	(d) Business
_____	11. support of well-baby clinics, youth recreation centers, and "scouts"	(e) Government
_____	12. increased literacy programs	
_____	13. a servant and tool of the majority of people	

Part III

Select and circle your choice of the best answer or answers for these statements:

14. A close alliance between nutrient need and physical development needs to be understood and stressed in nutrition education because:
    (a) the nutritional state of the individual is affected by his genetic pattern
    (b) all individuals regardless of age need the same kinds and amounts of nutrients
    (c) the age of the person has little effect upon the need for certain foods
    (d) the nutrient balance is crucial during the periods of most rapid growth
    (e) all of the above

15. The average weight of a child at birth is:
    (a) determined by genetics
    (b) partially dependent upon the nutrients supplied by the mother
    (c) unrelated to the state of health of the mother
    (d) increased by the consumption of protein by the mother throughout pregnancy
    (e) dependent upon the amount of weight gained by the mother during the first trimester

16. The growth of the human body proceeds in an orderly sequence of events and has certain indicators of maturation for a child which include:
    (a) body weight
    (b) diameter of wrist
    (c) length of arms
    (d) soft tissue development
    (e) carpal bone development

17. A ten-month-old child can feed himself certain foods such as:
    (a) oatmeal and pudding
    (b) carrot sticks and apple slices
    (c) ice cream and sherbet
    (d) applesauce and pureed peas
    (e) cooked meat and liver strips

18. Infants of all races during the first months of life are relatively well fed because:
    (a) a limited amount of food is consumed
    (b) few food choices are desired or required
    (c) milk is the universal diet of good quality
    (d) parental knowledge of infant needs is an influential factor
    (e) plenty of food is available for the infant

19. The nutritional status of preschool children may decrease because:
    (a) they frequently change their likes and dislikes for food

(b) they are disinterested in the kinds of food
(c) they are permitted to eat whatever they desire
(d) parents lack awareness and understanding of food needs
(e) all of the above

20. The ecology of human nutrition can be interpreted to mean:
    (a) methods in which the individual nutritional status is supported by education, business, good government, allied health, etc.
    (b) the interrelationship of the multiple facets of human endeavor
    (c) the mutual relationship between people and their environment
    (d) multiple areas of concern culminating in available food supplies and healthy individuals
    (e) all of the above

21. Height-weight-age ratios are *not* good criteria for judging growth and physical well-being because:
    (a) average measurements do not reflect individual variations in size
    (b) average measurement do not reflect individual's state of health
    (c) two individuals can weigh the same amount; yet one can be fat and the other normal weight
    (d) an athlete who is the same height and weight as a nonathlete will not have the same adiposity
    (e) all of the above

22. The most abundant component of the body other than water is:
    (a) fat
    (b) vitamins
    (c) protein
    (d) carbohydrate
    (e) minerals

23. If a person consumes 250 calories less than he needs each day, how long will it take to loose 5 pounds?
    (a) 4 weeks
    (b) 6 weeks
    (c) 8 weeks
    (d) 10 weeks
    (e) 12 weeks

24. Some characteristics of people who have inadequate food supplies have been discussed. From the following lists circle those terms which would be applicable to such people.

anemic	illiterate	robust
energetic	cheerful	stout
neat	edematous	mentally alert
apathetic	listless	skeletal malalignment

well-groomed	emaciated	fears, superstitions
vigorous	rejection	coordinated
weak	radiation	joyous
prideful	tired	nimble
phlegmatic	pale	happy
distended stomach	fatigued	

4

Dietary Specifications to Meet Nutritional Needs

What Devices Are Used to Plan and to Judge Adequacy of Dietary Intake?

We all eat; we are motivated to eat by many different stimuli which range from seeing the time on the clock, to meeting someone, to noting growling, uncomfortable feeling at the beltline. We eat for many reasons completely unrelated to the body's need for food. Do you think this is a good policy?

Not only do we eat without plan, but we also make the choice of food to eat by chance. Conscious planning for food to comprise the daily meals and snacks must take precedence as the simplest form of learning about applied nutrition. To aid in this learning, several food promotion organizations have designed schemes for planning meals which assure adequate food intake. You cannot go wrong as long as you use a systematic, conscious selection of food based on the nutrient requirements of the people involved.

A periodic computation of the nutrient content of this systematic, rational choice of food helps to assure the diner that his daily food intake meets the Recommended Dietary Allowances (RDA) as established by the Food and Nutrition Board of the National Research Council (NRC) in the United States.

EVERYDAY FOOD GUIDES TO NUTRITION

Objectives

1. To be aware of the efforts which have been made to define dietary needs as related to human well-being, e.g., food groups and the National Research Council's Recommended Dietary Allowances.
2. To recall that nutrients supplied by the diet are the fundamental bases for all growth and development.
3. To be familiar with the specific, quantitative nutrient needs of the average reference man and woman and with influences of age and pregnancy on nutrient need.

Food Guides — A Tool for Meal Planning

The science of nutrition, like other sciences, is complex. For practical use, nutritionists have devised a teaching tool — a food guide which translates knowledge of nutritional needs and nutrient content of food into a simple plan for directing food choices. By following such a guide, most persons can select a nutritionally adequate diet which satisfies their cultural, ethnic, and social concepts as well as their health needs.

Even though nutrition and food preparation are classed as sciences, relying heavily on chemistry and biology, the people involved in food processing and preparation relate food and nutrition to the behavioral and social sciences as well. Advertising stresses man's awareness of producing palatability in cookery, and eye-appeal in service of food must not be overlooked. Effort must be made to impress people that nutritious food, even though scientifically planned and produced, is planned for them personally, recognizing their values and concepts about food acceptance derived from traditionally and artistically created flavors and appearances. All too often a person considers nutrition a medical or pharmaceutical type science in conflict with his own desire, taste, and acceptance of "good food." Many jokes are centered on the concept that the food which a person prefers to eat is either sinful or fattening and that nutritious food is in conflict with tasty, desirable meals.

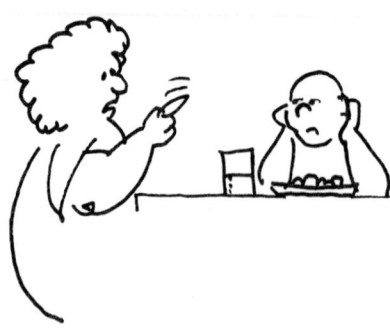

Fig. 4.1 Nagging can alienate the most receptive eater.

This image of conflict between desirable food and nutritious meals is undoubtedly created in the homes of a society which indulges in immediate pleasure with disregard for long-range satisfaction. The creative homemaker can develop the concept that "good food is also nutritious" when she prepares for birthday parties, rewards, and other special events. Why should dessert not be as nutritious as an entree, or a vegetable have as much appeal as a snack? The problem is partly the traditional image which has been created for specific food by a family and the social customs in a community. The other part of the problem is the thought and effort which is concentrated on so-called "reward and party" foods in contrast to those served in everyday meals.

Enough emphasis must be placed on the role the homemaker has in shaping the food acceptance of the family along the lines of meeting the physiological needs as well as those of a social, cultural, and aesthetic nature. Furthermore, the homemaker must realize that criticism, nagging, and repeated emphasis on nutritional quality can alienate the most receptive eater.

Regularity of eating several times a day is essential for adequate nutrient intake.

1. Children must be fed a balanced food intake from six to three times daily depending on age; adults can share this schedule but without excess consumption.
2. At each meal some food such as meat, milk, cheese, eggs, nuts, or products made from these should be included for people of all ages.
3. Children can select the food they prefer as long as "frill" foods are not available for competition in the choices.
4. Carefully selected foods save money in medical expenses and may result in good health for the child as well as for the adult or aged person.
5. Well-planned snack foods should be available for children to help themselves according to their appetite and activity schedule.

Needed food can be added to the family's favorite dishes, for example:

1. To ground meats for hamburgers and meat loaf, tomatoes, dried milk, eggs, chopped green onions, and celery tops, and chopped spinach, can be added depending on dietary need, but do not add everything every time!
2. To cooked beans, tomatoes, ham, beef, other meats, green onion, celery tops, or carrots can be added.
3. To any flour, cornmeal, masa, bread, or cereal product can be

added twice the milk in the recipe by use of dried milk, example: use $\frac{2}{3}$ cup dried milk and 1 cup water in place of 1 cup fresh milk, depending on dietary need involved.

4. To homemade breads made with whole wheat flour, yellow corn-meal, and enriched white flour, dried milk, eggs, and other nutritious foods can be added; these foods then are excellent between-meal foods, examples: chopped sausage, ham scraps, cheese, dried fruits, and nuts can be added to cornbread, biscuits, muffins, or pancakes.

Low-cost foods may be more nutritious than expensive ones as indicated in these contrasts:

1. Potatoes baked or boiled in peelings as compared to "instant" potatoes or potato chips.
2. Plain cheeses such as long-horn or processed American as com-pared to cheese spreads, cream cheese, and novelty specialties.
3. Homemade milk chocolate (dried milk, cocoa mix and either cold or hot water) compared with dairy-made or packaged drink.
4. Homemade cornmeal products compared with corn chips, frozen bread, or novelty items.
5. Chuck and shoulder beef or pork cuts instead of round or loin cuts; sausage and bacon with high fat cost as much as $2 to $3 per lb. for the portion eaten. Prices on many sandwich meats are also mislead-ing because often these are high in fat and water content.
6. Fresh milk should be used only for drinking and cheaper dried or canned milk is best when used in cooking and baking.
7. Price does not indicate quality or nutritive value of food items.

Variations of the food guides currently used as tools for teaching food selection in meal planning include the example in Fig. 4.2.

Food plans at different cost levels have been developed by the USDA as bases for planning nutritionally adequate diets for groups of families with varying amounts of money to spend for food. One plan for low-cost meals was published in 1969. This plan indicates the quantities of food needed in one week from each of the food groups to provide three meals at home every day for family members in different age-sex classifications. The food group quantities suggested in the food plan provide the servings outlined in the foundation diet of the Daily Food Guides and allow for food to "round out" meals, satisfy appetites, and complete the food energy and nutrient needs.

The low-cost food plans are designed for thrifty families that must

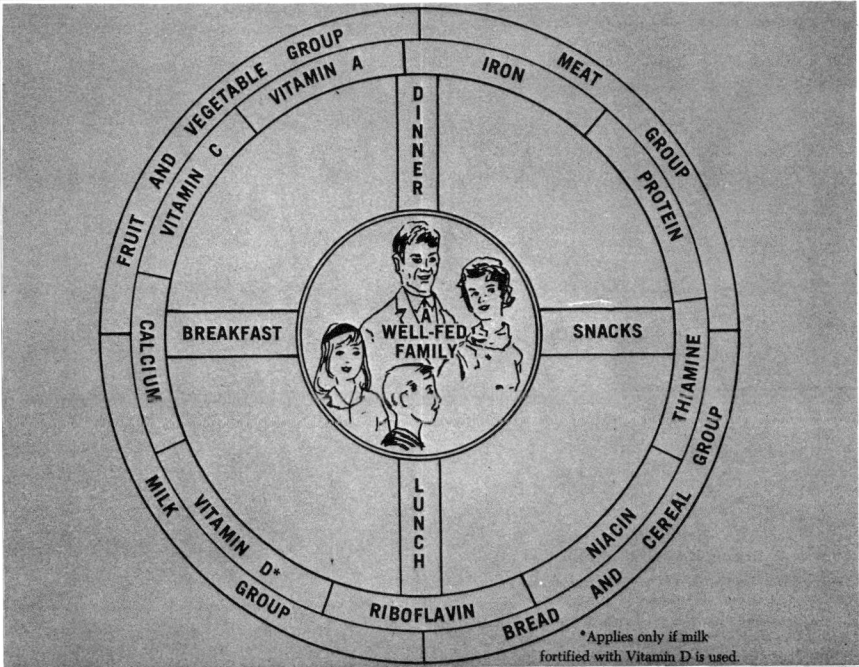

Fig. 4.2   HE Extension Leaflet No. 25. N.Y. State College of Human Ecology, Cornell University, Ithaca, New York.

buy all or most of their food. The designation "low-cost" is relative and may not represent the minimum cost at which nutritional needs can be met. The quantities of food planned are sufficient to allow for only a minimum of discard and plate waste beyond the normal loss of bone and inedible refuse. Menus based on this plan will not be elaborate as they must include low-cost foods that lack "built-in conveniences," require a considerable amount of home preparation, and call for skill in cooking to make varied and appetizing meals.

Trends in Dietary Habits

A survey of 7500 households in the spring of 1965 conducted by the U.S. Department of Agriculture Research showed that:

(a) on the average, amounts of food used in U.S. households were sufficient to provide diets that met the Recommended Dietary Allowances set by the NRC for calories, protein, for the mineral elements, calcium and iron; and for the vitamins, vitamin A value, thiamine, riboflavin, and ascorbic acid;

(b) half of the households had diets that met the allowances for all nutrients; and,

(c) the other half of the households had diets that failed to meet the allowances of one or more nutrients. Calcium, vitamin A value and ascorbic acid were the nutrients most often below the allowances.

Gortner (1970) of the U.S. Department of Agriculture reported in "Forums in Focus" that recent trends in the food consumption patterns are toward greater consumption of meat and certain dairy products, a lowered consumption of potatoes and many cereal products, and an increased portion of total calories coming from fat. A special survey of 50,000 United States college students showed that liver was the most disliked food and that vegetables and salads were not particularly liked. The best-liked foods were beef, potatoes, bread, and desserts. Also, a strong tendency toward avoiding high calorie foods was shown by the girls who participated in the survey. Results of this survey caused concern about the adequacy of the diets in the United States especially for adequate amounts of calcium and iron for young females.

Probably more persons in the United States are malnourished because of misinformation, ignorance, and indifference about nutrition than because of poverty. The following diary is, of course, an exaggeration, but the conditions described probably exist more often than either the general public or the food industry would care to admit.

The Diary of a Schoolgirl's Stomach

8:00 a.m.—Oh dear! Another cold day. I wonder if she will expect me to supply warmth today on the same rations I've been getting lately. Got up too late for breakfast and had to run for the bus.

9:00 a.m.—It is time for "gum" and no food yet. I wonder if she thinks I can run forever on no food.

10:30 a.m.—All heated up to the boiling point—those were terrible exercises for me to bear on my emptiness. Two glasses of ice water just arrived, the shock has almost paralyzed me.

10:40 a.m.—No class this period. Thought I'd get breakfast, but two candy bars arrived instead. Both were brain food. I wish I could send them to her head. Now a continual stream of peanuts are coming. More ice water.

11:00 a.m.—Peanuts keep drifting along. Think she has finished them now.

12:00 noon—Decided she was not very hungry so instead of a good hot solid lunch she sent down a hamburger sandwich and a chocolate malt. Could have managed it if it just had not been quite so rich and only half chewed.

12:30 p.m.—More ice water.

1:00 p.m. – Hope she gives me an hour or two of complete rest now. Oh horrors! She has found another handful of peanuts in her pocket.

1:30 p.m. – Her girlfriend just handed her an apple. Just heard her say she was sure the malted milk must have been sour.

2:30 p.m. – A guy in tortoise shell rimmed glasses just remembered he owed her a treat so they walked over to the store on the corner and bought 20¢ worth of jelly beans.

3:30 p.m. – Defeated at a game of tennis and had to treat her opponent. Mercy! It was chili with accent on the pepper. More ice water.

4:30 p.m. – Bromo Seltzer arrives.

5:30 p.m. – Mad dash for the car.

6:00 p.m. – Supper finally. Boiled cabbage, fried potatoes, pork chops, pickles, and banana cream pie. This is impossible.

7:30 p.m. – A headache, and it's time to go to the freshmen character ball. Oh no! Here come the aspirin.

11:00 p.m. – Refreshments at the ball – gobs of ice cream and cake. Just heard her say, "Bob, I don't feel well, let's hurry home."

11:30 p.m. – Sent back the ice cream and cake.

11:40 p.m. – Just sent back the banana pie.

12:00 midnight – Cabbage, chops, potatoes and pickles expelled.

12:15 a.m. – Hasty call for the Doctor!

12:30 a.m. – Doctor says she is subject to nervous stomach. Her mother says it's something she inherited from her father and daughter declares that her school work is just too hard for her.

Author Unknown

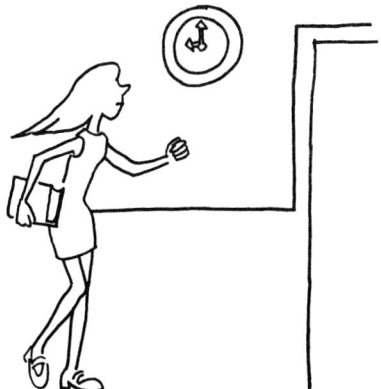

Fig. 4.3   Got up too late for breakfast.

Activities for Student Learning

1. You need to design a daily food intake for a multimeal and snack schedule for a young person such as you, listing time of day and the amount of food you would eat.
2. Continuing with the same design, suppose that a hard working husband who sits at a desk most of the day and watches TV at night, a four-year-old preschool child, and a seven-year-old school child were in this family, you need to adjust the design of the day's food to include the needs and preferences of these persons, knowing the husband and the school child eat lunch away from home.
3. Review the kind of dietary habits that are reflected by the "The Diary of a Schoolgirl's Stomach."
4. Indicate how the smaller amounts eaten by the children can be fortified in order to meet their dietary needs without raising the calorie content of the meals for the adults; use some of the suggested food sources for supplementation for the nutrients that are needed.
5. You will want to plan a week's menus for a young adult like yourself whether you eat in the dormitory cafeteria or at home.
6. Remember:

Hot Tips:

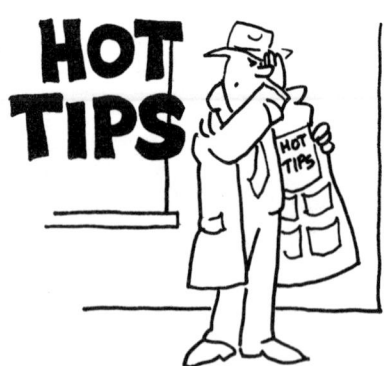

New Words:

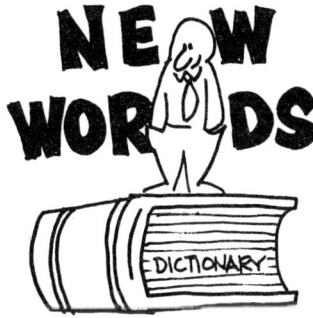

RECOMMENDED DIETARY ALLOWANCES

Objectives

1. To identify the biochemical research that defines nutrition in terms of chemical units called nutrients.
2. To realize that as knowledge of nutrients increases, adjustments will need to be made in the amounts of nutrients recommended to be eaten by various individuals.

Development of Dietary Recommendations

Even prior to 1940, Henry C. Sherman, formerly professor of chemistry and nutrition at Columbia University, was greatly concerned about the relation of dietary intake and nutritional status; he worked toward the establishment of quantitative levels of nutrient consumption to assure well-being. Before the chemical formula for any vitamin was determined, Sherman attempted to standardize the measurement in terms of either the amount of rat-growth or the degree of cure of typical deficiency symptoms in the rat resulting from a certain quantity of food. These amounts were referred to as "rat units" to indicate the potency of a food as a source of a given vitamin. Mary S. Rose, who was highly concerned about nutrition education, set up standards in terms of shares, 30 shares being the amount needed by the average adult man and everyone else requiring fewer or more shares. Even now, references are made to "man units" of food as a basis for calculating dietary needs of people the world over.

Finally, under the pressure of urgency inflicted by World War II, the National Research Council's Food and Nutrition Board issued, in 1941, the Recommended Dietary Allowances under the assumption that the amounts would be modified from time to time as the Board reviewed the most recent research on nutritional needs of people. The 1968 revision is shown in Table 4.1.

The concept used by the Board was that the minimum amount of a nutrient required to prevent symptoms of deficiency should be supplemented by a "margin for safety" in order to derive a recommended dietary allowance. The "margin for safety" was defined as a quantity of intake which would allow for natural variations in the concentration of a nutrient in food or the ease with which it may be lost in preparation and service; and second, would allow for variation in an individual person's utilization and bodily need for that nutrient. As a result, the "margin for safety" differed for each of the nutrients for which dietary recommendations had been determined.

For most individuals an intake of 75% of the RDA may be safe but more risk is involved than when the intake is 100%. Recommendations for intake of calories were not included, since the level of activity of people is highly variable and adequacy of calorie intake for adults can be judged easily by constancy of weight. Table 4.2 shows comparisons of different recommendations for nutrient intakes for the average man and woman.

Activities for Student Learning

1. You should be able to describe the background which probably led to the establishment of a nationwide standardization of recommended nutrient intakes.

2. When you study the table on Recommended Dietary Allowances, note changes which occur with age; choose one nutrient and make a bar graph to show the total amount of that nutrient which is recommended for each age interval; make a second graph which compares the amount recommended per kilogram body weight for each age interval.

3. Summarize the changes in recommended amounts of nutrients which have been made in the last several revisions of the Recommended Dietary Allowances (RDA), for example, those made in 1958, 1963, and 1968.

Table 4.1 Food and Nutrition Board, National Academy of Sciences—National Research Council (Recommended Daily Dietary Allowances) (Revised 1968 Designed for the maintenance of good nutrition of practically all healthy people in the U.S.A.).

	Age[2] Years From Up to	Weight Kg (lbs)	Height cm (in.)	Kcal	Protein g	Vitamin A Activity IU	Vitamin D Activity IU	Vitamin E Activity IU	Ascorbic Acid mg	Folacin[3] mg	Niacin mg equiv.[4]	Riboflavin mg	Thiamine mg	Vitamin B6 mg	Vitamin B12 μg	Calcium g	Phosphorus g	Iodine μg	Iron mg	Magnesium mg
Infants	0–1/6	4 (9)	55 22	kg × 120	kg × 2.2[5]	1500	400	5	35	0.05	5	0.4	0.2	0.2	1.0	0.4	0.2	25	6	40
	1/6–1/2	7 (15)	63 25	kg × 110	kg × 2.0[5]	1500	400	5	35	0.05	7	0.5	0.4	0.3	1.5	0.5	0.4	40	10	60
	1/2–1	9 (20)	72 28	kg × 100	kg × 1.8[5]	1500	400	5	35	0.1	8	0.6	0.5	0.4	2.0	0.6	0.5	45	15	70
Children	1–2	12 (26)	81 32	1100	25	2000	400	10	40	0.1	8	0.6	0.6	0.5	2.0	0.7	0.7	55	15	100
	2–3	14 (31)	91 36	1250	25	2000	400	10	40	0.2	8	0.7	0.6	0.6	2.5	0.8	0.8	60	15	150
	3–4	16 (35)	100 39	1400	30	2500	400	10	40	0.2	9	0.8	0.7	0.7	3	0.8	0.8	70	10	200
	4–6	19 (42)	110 43	1600	30	2500	400	10	40	0.2	11	0.9	0.8	0.9	4	0.8	0.8	80	10	200
	6–8	23 (51)	121 48	2000	35	3500	400	15	40	0.2	13	1.1	1.0	1.0	4	0.9	0.9	100	10	250
	8–10	28 (62)	131 52	2200	40	3500	400	15	40	0.3	15	1.2	1.1	1.2	5	1.0	1.0	110	10	250
Males	10–12	35 (77)	140 55	2500	45	4500	400	20	40	0.4	17	1.3	1.3	1.4	5	1.2	1.2	125	10	300
	12–14	43 (95)	151 59	2700	50	5000	400	20	45	0.4	18	1.4	1.4	1.6	5	1.4	1.4	135	18	350
	14–18	59 (130)	170 67	3000	60	5000	400	25	55	0.4	20	1.5	1.5	1.8	5	1.4	1.4	150	18	400
	18–22	67 (147)	175 69	2800	60	5000	400	30	60	0.4	18	1.6	1.4	2.0	5	0.8	0.8	140	10	400
	22–35	70 (154)	175 69	2800	65	5000	—	30	60	0.4	18	1.7	1.4	2.0	5	0.8	0.8	140	10	350
	35–55	70 (154)	173 68	2600	65	5000	—	30	60	0.4	17	1.7	1.3	2.0	5	0.8	0.8	125	10	350
	55–75+	70 (154)	171 67	2400	65	5000	—	30	60	0.4	14	1.7	1.2	2.0	6	0.8	0.8	110	10	350
Females	10–12	35 (77)	142 56	2250	50	4500	400	20	40	0.4	15	1.3	1.1	1.4	5	1.2	1.2	110	18	300
	12–14	44 (97)	154 61	2300	50	5000	400	20	45	0.4	15	1.4	1.2	1.6	5	1.3	1.3	115	18	350
	14–16	52 (114)	157 62	2400	55	5000	400	25	50	0.4	16	1.4	1.2	1.8	5	1.3	1.3	120	18	350
	16–18	54 (119)	160 63	2300	55	5000	400	25	50	0.4	15	1.5	1.2	2.0	5	1.3	1.3	115	18	350
	18–22	58 (128)	163 64	2000	55	5000	400	25	55	0.4	13	1.5	1.0	2.0	5	0.8	0.8	100	18	350
	22–35	58 (128)	163 64	2000	55	5000	—	25	55	0.4	13	1.5	1.0	2.0	5	0.8	0.8	100	18	300
	35–55	58 (128)	160 63	1850	55	5000	—	25	55	0.4	13	1.5	1.0	2.0	5	0.8	0.8	90	18	300
	55–75+	58 (128)	157 62	1700	55	5000	—	25	55	0.4	13	1.5	1.0	2.0	6	0.8	0.8	80	10	300
Pregnancy				+200	65	6000	400	30	60	0.8	15	1.8	+0.1	2.5	8	+0.4	+0.4	125	18	450
Lactation				+1000	75	8000	400	30	60	0.5	20	2.0	+0.5	2.5	6	+0.5	+0.5	150	18	450

[1]The allowance levels are intended to cover individual variations among most normal persons as they live in the United States under usual environmental stresses. The recommended allowances can be attained with a variety of common foods, providing other nutrients for which human requirements have been less well defined. See text for more detailed discussion of allowances and of nutrients not tabulated.

[2]Entries on lines for age range 22–35 years represent the reference man and woman at age 22. All other entries represent allowances for the midpoint of the specified age range.

[3]The folacin allowances refer to dietary sources as determined by *Lactobacillus casei* assay. Pure forms of folacin may be effective in doses less than 1/4 of the RDA.

[4]Niacin equivalents include dietary sources of the vitamin itself plus 1 mg equivalent for each 60 mg of dietary tryptophan.

[5]Assumes protein equivalent to human milk. For proteins not 100 percent utilized factors should be increased proportionately.

71

Table 4.2   Comparison of different recommendations for nutrient intakes for the average man and woman.

Nutrient		NRC's RDA[1] 1968 Man– Woman	U.S. Recommended Daily Allowances for Nutrition Labeling 1973[2]	Dietary Standards	
				Canadian[3] 1964 Man– Woman	British[4] Man– Woman
Protein	g	65–55	45–65	50–39	66–58
Calcium	mg	800	1000	500	800
Iron	mg	10–18	18	6–10	12
Vitamin A	IU	5000	5000	3700	5000
Thiamine	mg	1.4–1.0	1.5	0.9–0.7	0.9–0.8
Riboflavin	mg	1.7–1.5	1.7	1.4–1.2	1.4–1.2
Niacin Equiv.	mg	18–13	20	9.0–7.0	9.8
Ascorbic Acid	mg	60–55	60	30	20

[1]Recommended Dietary Allowances 7th ed., 1968. National Academy Sciences, Washington, D.C.

[2]For adults and children of 4 or more years of age; 45 g for high quality, 65 g for general proteins

[3]Dietary Standards for Canada, Canadian Bull. Nutrition 6,1, 1964. Dept. of Public Printing and Stationery, Ottawa.

[4]Committee on Nutrition, British Medical Association, 1950.

NUTRIENT CONTENT OF FOOD

Objectives

1. To recognize that food as produced by agriculture, processed, stored, and transported by industry is not a stable commodity.
2. To manipulate food in order to retain its nutrient content during preparation with the possible exception of fat content of meats and foods cooked in fat.
3. To demonstrate the methods by which nutrients can be added during food preparation through the use of selected ingredients.
4. To accept that the responsibility is on the individual when he eats away from home, both in selection of a place in which to eat and in the safety and quality of the food chosen.

Retention of Nutrients

Sarcasm and jokes are directed to the housewife who is said "to throw out more in garbage at the back door than the husband can bring home through the front." Or that "the best fed member of the family is the sink and garbage disposal unit."

Some of the pitfalls of nutrient losses from food are outlined for consideration:

I. Solubility in water is the greatest single factor causing loss of nutrients during food preparation.

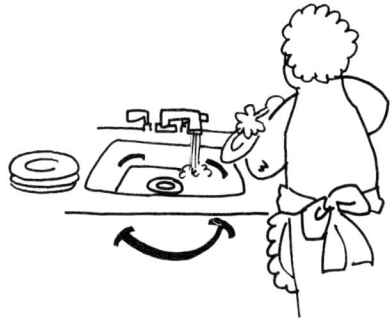

Fig. 4.4 The best fed member of the family is the sink garbage disposal unit.

A. Juices from canned foods are relatively high in water soluble nutrients, namely, the water soluble vitamins and mineral elements.
   1. From $\frac{1}{3}$ to $\frac{1}{2}$ of the mineral content of a food is in the juice of canned food.
   2. About $\frac{1}{2}$ of the water soluble vitamin content of a can of food is in the juice.
   3. The amount dissolved in the juice of any one item depends on:
      (a) The soundness and toughness of peelings.
      (b) The size of the pieces and the direction of cutting.
      (c) The consistency of the food, whether firm or mushy.

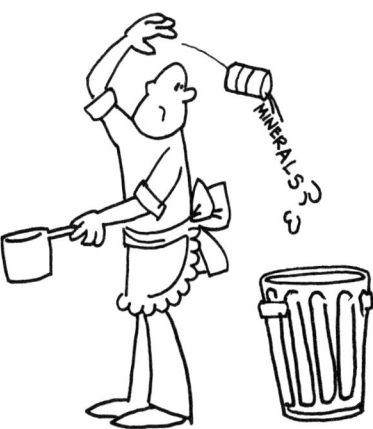

Fig. 4.5 About half of the mineral content is in the juice.

B. In fresh foods the amount of water used to cook is most significant, as well as the use made of the water left after the food is done. Factors to determine the amount of solution occurring while cooking in water include:
   1. The amount of water used in relation to the volume of food.
   2. Whether the food is peeled or not and how it is cut—small or large pieces and the direction of the cut.
   3. The length of time the food is in contact with water; fast cooking is recommended and accomplished by:

        (a) Covering the pan while the food is cooking to shorten cooking time.

        (b) Starting the food to cook in boiling water.

        (c) Using a pan size related to the burner or surface unit size.

        (d) Quality of the pan in relation to the rapidity of cooking —light-weight cheap pans with poorly fitting lids increase cooking time, supply irregular heat, and require more water with the food for cooking.

    4. Nutrients do not evaporate but some change chemically which causes a loss of potency and others dissolve.

C. Soaking food in water for any one of a number of reasons may seriously affect the nutrient content unless the soaking water is utilized.

    1. The soaking water from dried fruits and legumes should be used as a cooking medium for that food.

    2. Foods prepared ahead of time should not be left standing in water until used. Some foods should not be prepared ahead and others can be stored more efficiently in covered containers or moisture-proof wraps.

    3. Freshening a wilted food should be done before the food is cut; better yet—vegetables and fruits should never be allowed to wilt.

    4. Blanching in steam is superior to water-bath for reduction of solution losses; parboiling is an outmoded process in that some of the water soluble nutrients are discarded.

D. Frozen foods can be very high in nutrient retention:

    1. Greatest losses in freezing foods occur in improper blanching—too long a period and using water rather than steam.

    2. Frozen food should be thawed a minimum amount, if at all, prior to cooking. Thawing should be done only in order to separate pieces. If juices drain, these should be used with the food.

    3. The freezing process itself has no detrimental effect unless improper temperatures are used. A temperature below 0°F is essential for nutrient retention, quality control, and the keeping qualities of the food.

    4. Packaging to exclude air, retain moisture, and prevent damage to food in frozen storage is essential.

5. Temperature control during storage at zero, or below, is also vital.

II. Certain vitamins are readily destroyed by heat (namely, thiamine, and ascorbic acid). This is a chemical decomposition related to the structure of the molecule; the term "kill vitamins" is therefore incorrect since vitamins are not living organisms.

   A. Increased temperature is more destructive than increased cooking time. Cooking is often a balance between time, temperature, and size of pieces which must all be considered together.

     1. Pressure cooking can be especially damaging if time is not carefully controlled as related to size pieces.

     2. Dry heat decomposes thiamine more readily than moist; therefore, toasting and browning decrease retention.

     3. The greater the surface area exposed to dry heat, the less the retention of nutrients as compared with cooking in larger pieces, for example, rolls as compared with a loaf of bread, or ground meat compared to roast.

     4. Thermostatically or thermometer controlled frying causes very little nutrient decomposition by heat; the absence of water also aids in unusually high retention values; fat soluble vitamins do not dissolve into the cooking fat.

   B. Longer cooking times at higher temperatures greatly increase decomposition.

   C. The presence of both air and heat is more detrimental than either alone. Air incorporated into hot foods as whipped potatoes may destroy all the ascorbic acid present in the original food.

   D. High temperature during storage can be very detrimental, such as storerooms above 60°F and refrigerators above 40°F.

III. Decomposition of vitamins by alkali may become significant.

   A. Use of baking soda (sodium bicarbonate) may reduce the ascorbic acid and thiamine content of various foods, for instance:

     1. Use of soda to neutralize the acidity of tomatoes in making cream of tomato soup must be avoided.

    2. To use soda with green vegetables to maintain green color is most undesirable.

    3. To tenderize dried beans by the use of a very small amount of soda added to the water for soaking beans for one hour is acceptable provided that this water is then discarded, the beans rinsed and soaked in fresh water which will be used in the cooking.

  B. The use of soda in flour mixtures is more destructive than that of baking powder which is a buffered product.

    1. Soda has been traditionally used with buttermilk, molasses, and other acid foods. Today's buttermilk has an extremely low acidity which requires only $\frac{1}{4}$ tsp. soda per cup of milk; old recipes need adjustment.

    2. Yeast produces an acid medium which is very good for retention of nutrients in baked foods.

IV. Influence of ultraviolet light on riboflavin is such that its exposure on both food and on people must be carefully controlled. This control also applies to sunlight which is a natural source of ultraviolet radiation.

V. Conditions which might result in excessive nutrient loss from food:

  A. Commercial food production with use of excess water, soda, and poor preparation practices; also, excessive time for holding food on steam tables.

  B. Eating at odd times several hours after food was prepared (haphazard meal schedule).

  C. Improper storage of food allowing wilting, deterioration at high temperatures (above 40°F), storage in water, exposure of cut surfaces to air and warm temperatures.

  D. Frozen foods which were partially thawed and then refrozen.

Fortification of Food at Home

Times occur in every person's life when either food consumption is reduced or the dietary need for nutrients is increased. A person knowledgeable in food and its composition can manipulate a diet by controlling the ingredients used in the food served. Examples of situations when the composition of a diet may be of special concern include:

1. conditions of stress especially for children and adolescents which interfere with either desire to eat or time required for meals,
2. during illness and convalescence when appetite lags and normal volume of intake is intolerable,
3. during last trimester of pregnancy when calorie restriction and lack of space in the abdomen make regular size meals impractical,
4. in the aged a lack of interest and tolerance of food often limits food intake in amount and variety.

Food can be fortified in the kitchen at home. The type of fortification should depend on which nutrients or which food may be needed by the individual or if general improvement is indicated with or without extra calories.

Suppose the dietary problems turn out to be an attitude of "drinking no milk" on the part of a child on a binge or of grandmother who is in a wheelchair recuperating from a fractured hip. Nonfat dried milk (NFD milk) is a real asset in such situations. Normally this milk would be added with the dry ingredients in a recipe; reconstitution is required only when a beverage is desired, then follow directions on the package. The NFD milk can be added either in addition to fresh milk specified in the recipe, to recipes in which no milk is specified, or in place of the regular milk using water for the volume of liquid required. Since different brands of NFD milk vary in the volume required to be equivalent to one cup or one quart of fresh milk, the recommendation on the package should be used. In most cases twice the amount specified in proportion to the liquid can be used. Added NFD milk increases protein, calcium, and B-vitamins of the food involved.

In summary, more milk can be used in meals:

To fluid milk and milk beverages, add $\frac{1}{4}$ cup of NFD milk for each cup of liquid.

To soups, add $\frac{1}{4}$–$\frac{1}{2}$ cup NFD milk for each cup of liquid.

To main dishes, add $\frac{1}{2}$ cup of NFD milk for every 4–6 servings to the ingredients in the recipes. Use in

Meat loaf	Creamed eggs
Spanish omelet	Cheese fondue
Macaroni and cheese	Welsh rarebit

To cream sauces and gravies, add $\frac{1}{4}$ cup NFD milk for each cup of fluid called for in the recipe.

To breads, biscuits, waffles, and griddle cakes, add $\frac{1}{4}$ cup NFD milk for each cup fluid called for in the recipe.

To cooked cereals, add $\frac{1}{2}$–1 cup NFD milk for every six servings being prepared. Cook over a low heat.

To recipes for puddings, custards, cookies, and cakes, add from $\frac{1}{2}$–$\frac{3}{4}$ cup NFD milk for every family-size recipe.

Selected foods are unusually potent sources of certain nutrients and could serve to fortify a diet in need of greater amounts. Such fortification is strictly a matter of choosing the appropriate food to be added to a regular diet or to a particular dish in a meal. Such a food should not increase the amount of food eaten or change its calorie content, since it is a substitute or adds neglible amount. Since vitamins A and C and iron are often low in dietaries, these can be supplied in increased amounts by incorporating the following foods into the diet, Tables 4.3 and 4.4.

A person needs to consider which of these foods can be substituted for less potent source of nutrients; e.g., the use of molasses instead of syrup, brown sugar in place of white as sources of iron in flour products and desserts.

At times, diets need to be fortified with protein of high biological value. The protein value of NFD milk has already been presented as 25 g per 1 C (70 g) of "instant" type NFD milk solids. Thus if $\frac{1}{4}$ C is added to an 8 oz beverage or 8 oz serving of soup or pudding, the protein content is increased by 6 g per serving over that in the regular recipe. Some interesting protein concentrates are available; these are

Table 4.3   Vitamin A values in selected foods.

For Vitamin A Value (5000 IU daily)*

Food	Amount	Vitamin A Value (IU)	Use in Menu
Apricots	1 (12/lb)	960	Snack, salad, dessert, preserves
Cantaloupe	$\frac{1}{4}$–5 in. dia.	3270	Snack, salad, dessert
Carrot	1–5 in. long	5500	Snack, salad, coke or cookies, cooked
Liver	1 oz cooked	15,140	Snack, meat loaf, sandwich filling
Parsley	1 Tbsp. chopped	300	Salad, meats, gravy, sandwiches
"Greens"	$\frac{1}{4}$ C cooked	2283	Salad, sandwiches, cooked

*Values from Handbook 8.

Table 4.4   Vitamin C and iron values in selected foods.

For Vitamin C (60 mg daily)*

Food	Amount	Ascorbic Acid (mg)	Use in Menu
Broccoli	¼ C cooked	34	Salad, vegetable, casserole
Cantaloupe	¼–5 in. dia.	32	Snack, salad, dessert
Cauliflower	¼ C cooked or raw	16	Salad, vegetable
Grapefruit	¼ C sections	18	Snack, salad, dessert
	¼ C juice	23	Punch, beverage
"Greens"	¼ C cooked	17	Salad, vegetable
Lemon/lime	2 Tbsp. juice	14/10	Tea, punch, salad, sauces, dessert
Orange	¼ C sections	30	Snack, salad, dessert
	¼ C juice	40	Beverage, punch
Peppers	1 oz ½ pod	63	Salad, with meats sauces
Strawberry	1 med. fresh	10	Snack, topping, dessert
Tomato	1 (3/lb)	34	Salad, vegetable
	¼ C canned	10	

For Iron (10–18 mg daily)*

Food	Amount	Iron (mg)	Use in Menu
Almond	¼ C	1.7	Snacks, salads, vegetables, desserts
Apricots	10 halves	2.1	Snack, salad, accompany meats, desserts, preserves
Beans, dry	½ C cooked	2.5	Salad, vegetable, casserole, entree
Beef, lean	3 oz cooked	3.3	Snack, salad, sandwiches, entree
Bread, enriched	2 sl.	1.2	Multiple uses
Chili con carne with beans	½ C cooked	2.1	Entree
Liver	2 oz cooked	5.0	Snack; sandwiches, casserole, entree
Molasses, light	2 Tbsp.	1.8	Ingredient in many products
Peas, green	½ C canned	2.1	Soups, salads, vegetable, casserole
Pork, lean	3 oz cooked	3.0	Snack, sandwiches, salad, entree
Prune juice	½ C	5.3	Beverage, desserts
Sugar, brown	2 Tbsp.	1.0	Ingredient in many products

*Values from Handbook 8.

identified in advertisements in current issues of the dietetic, hospital, and medical journals.

Favorite recipes for many food products can be fortified to furnish extra nutrients. In many cases, such fortification not only increases the nutrient content but can become a creative project of using "leftovers" and "tag ends" such as different flours, peanut butter, nuts, raisins, etc. Thus a wise practice is developed which can result in saving money on the grocery bill and in the decreased consumption of "empty calorie" foods. An example of fortification in which the nutrient content of protein, calcium, iron, and vitamin A was increased is shown in the following recipe.

FORTY-EIGHT FORTIFIED OAT AND LASSES NUGGETS

1¼ C brown sugar creamed with 1 C margarine at room temperature.

Add 2 eggs, beat well.

Mix together:

> 1½ C enriched flour
> 2 tsp. baking powder
> ½ C NFD milk solids
> 1 tsp. cinnamon (if desired)

Add about ½ of the dry mix to egg, sugar, and fat mixture, and blend well.

Add ½ C heavy molasses, the rest of the dry mix, and blend well.

Stir in 3–4 C quick cooking rolled oats. Mix until all oatflakes are no longer white. Add enough oats to make a stiff, firm mass which will not drop from a teaspoon.

Add 1 C more or less of any kind of nuts and of dried fruit such as raisins, chopped prunes, figs, etc.

Drop in mounds the size of a pecan on lightly oiled baking sheets. Bake for 12–15 minutes in a 400°F oven. The dough should spread very little during baking. If it does spread flat, add more oats to make it stiffer so that the baked product looks like nuggets and not flat wafers.

Additional recipes illustrating food fortification to increase nutrient content are:

Basic Biscuit Recipe
  1 C flour
  1½ tsp. baking powder
  3 Tbsp. margarine or butter
  ½ tsp. salt
  ⅓–½ C liquid (use water, fruit or vegetable juices such as orange, tomato, or other)
  ¼–½ C NFD milk solids and combine with flour

Mix according to directions for regular biscuits. Yield: 4 large or 8 small biscuits.

Basic Muffin Recipe
  1 C flour
  1¼ tsp. baking powder
  3 Tbsp. margarine or butter
  1 Tbsp. sugar (more may be used to make them more cake-like)
  1 egg
  ¼ tsp. salt

$\frac{1}{2}$ C liquid
$\frac{1}{4}$–$\frac{1}{2}$ C milk solids

Mix only enough to moisten, leaving batter rough and lumpy when putting into pans. Yields: 4 large or 8 small muffins.

For variety:
1. Use of brown sugar or molasses instead of pure white sugar adds flavor, calcium, and iron to any recipe.
2. Use $\frac{1}{2}$ of the flour and add equal amounts of whole wheat flour or whole wheat cereal such as rolled wheat or yellow cornmeal: use $\frac{1}{2}$ C liquid per cup if a mixture of flour and other cereal is used.
3. Add to either recipe $\frac{1}{4}$ C grated cheese; or $\frac{1}{4}$ C peanut butter; or $\frac{1}{4}$–$\frac{1}{2}$ C chopped ham or leftover cooked bacon.
4. When using fruit juices, use 2 Tbsp. brown sugar and about $\frac{1}{2}$ C of a mashed fruit such as canned or stewed apricots, prunes, bananas, dates, chopped or ground raisins, grated raw carrots, etc.
5. With biscuit dough, the added fruits, meats, cheese or peanut butter may be added as in making cinnamon rolls; roll dough $\frac{1}{2}$-in. thick, spread with "filling," roll up tightly. This may be baked whole and then sliced and served or it may be cut across about $\frac{1}{2}$-in. thick and baked in individual rolls close together in a pan or in a muffin pan with one roll per muffin cup.

Fortified Cornbread
1 C cornmeal plus $\frac{1}{4}$ C flour
1 tsp. baking powder
1 egg (could use 2 eggs)
$\frac{1}{2}$ tsp. salt
2 Tbsp. fat (bacon, ham drippings or 3 Tbsp. margarine)
$\frac{1}{3}$ C NFD milk solids
$\frac{1}{2}$–$\frac{2}{3}$ C liquid (water or vegetable juices)

Mix by same procedure as muffins. Yield: 4 large or 8 small muffins.

For variety:
1. Add $\frac{1}{2}$ lb cooked chili meat or 1 C dried ham or 4 sliced weiners or $\frac{1}{2}$ C cubed cheese.
2. Add $\frac{1}{2}$ C chopped green onions or olives or green peppers.
3. Add 1 C whole corn with green pepper or pimento or 1 C Mexicorn.
4. Use 1 C diced cooked carrots or 1 C grated raw carrot.
5. Use tomato juice as the liquid to add flavor, color, and food value.

Fortified Hot Cakes	*Syrup for Hot Cakes*
1 C water	1 lb dark brown sugar
1 egg	1 C water or canned fruit juice
2 Tbsp. oil	
1 C flour	Boil sugar in a portion of water to dissolve it; add flavoring and butter if desired.
$\frac{1}{2}$ C NFD milk solids	
1$\frac{1}{2}$ tsp. baking powder	
$\frac{1}{2}$ C oatmeal or rolled wheat	
3 Tbsp. yellow cornmeal	
1 tsp. salt	
2 tsp. sugar	

Hamburger or Ground Meat Dishes
Whether you make patties, hamburgers, or meat loaf, the following foods can be
added *per pound of meat*:
1. Add ½ C NFD milk solids plus ¼ C liquid (vegetable juice, water or meat
   broth). If meat is to be fried, do not add the milk because it will cause the
   meat to stick to the pan.
2. Use 1–2 eggs in addition to the dried milk.
3. Add 2–4 oz of liver, lightly fried in oil and then ground along with ¼ C of
   onions, ½ C of tomato juice, and 1 C of breadcrumbs.
4. Add any whole wheat cereal along with some liquid.
5. Use chopped parsley, carrots, onions, and tomatoes in any combination
   suited to the taste.

The Role of Dietary Supplements in Nutrition

Occasions arise when the volume of food eaten or the assortment
chosen from the food groups is limited. Such occasions or conditions
are outlined along with suggested procedures which can be used for
correction:

I. Conditions which may warrant a dietary supplement:

   A. Period of chronic illness, disease, or convalescence.
      1. Series of infections, especially in children or the aged.
      2. Organic disturbance as surgery, etc.
      3. Recovery from an accident involving bodily injury.

   B. Pregnancy and lactation.
      1. Last trimester may require added nutrients if calorie in-
         take is restricted, especially iron and possibly other
         nutrients.
      2. Success of lactation depends largely on adequate nutrient
         intake during pregnancy and lactation.

   C. Occupational strain, especially one with limited calorie ex-
      penditure and high responsibility.

   D. Period when emotional involvement interferes with regular
      meals and normal food intake.

II. Kind of nutrient concentrate to consider:

   A. Consult doctor who knows the particular situation.

   B. Consider what the dietary may be lacking — usually nutrients
      come in groups — for example:

1. Lack of milk in diet requires a supplement including protein, calcium, phosphorus, riboflavin and others.
2. Lack of fresh and raw fruits and vegetables requires a supplement of ascorbic acid and maybe vitamin A.

C. A nonchemical concentrate made from a natural food will furnish needed nutrients in acceptable proportions and also unidentified substances of possible physiological value.
   1. Yeast concentrates, including torula yeast, have a high potential in dietary supplementation.
   2. Nonfat dried milk has many dietary uses and a high nutrient content.
   3. Use of citrus fruit concentrates, in partially diluted form, furnishes certain nutrients in abundant supply.
   4. Liver from any animal furnishes an excellent means by which to fortify a diet with many nutrients.

III. Rules to observe in diet supplementation:

A. One should be sure that supplementation is needed and not just add more of the nutrients already consumed in abundance.

B. All supplements should be eaten in regular meals periodically throughout the day for best use of nutrients by the body tissues.

C. Small portions taken in balanced assortment of all nutrients at short intervals give better response than massive dosage taken once daily.

IV. Caution about excessive nutrient consumption:

A. Excessive intake of many substances changes an essential ingredient into a toxic one.
   1. Fluorine – 1 part per million is essential for hard, decay-resistant tooth enamel; over 2 parts per million causes dental fluorosis (mottled enamel).
   2. Vitamin A – 5000 IU is essential, whereas 50,000 IU taken for over several weeks may result in symptoms of serious toxicity.

B. Nutrients of which excessive amounts are not readily excreted may prove damaging to the very body tissues being treated.

1. Protein intakes twice the amounts recommended for children can cause serious damage in growth and normal development.
2. Fat-soluble vitamin accumulation in the liver and kidney may cause tissue damage.
3. Calorie intake in excess to energy needs accumulates in unsightly fat and is an increased hazard to successful aging.

C. Nutrition is achieved by a careful balance of nutrient intake. The balance can be easily upset and developed into gross deficiencies whenever one or more nutrients are consumed in massive amounts. Because abnormally large intakes (those in excess of the amount specified in RDA) of a few nutrients, or of many, distorts the balance of all dietary components to a degree, the body suffers rather than benefits from the supplementation.

Trends to Eat Food Away From Home

The change in society of the United States from rural to urban has introduced a number of alterations in eating habits. The major ones which greatly affect the nutritional status include:

1. Quick, ready-to-eat food items — purchased in vending machines or over the counter — may constitute a meal in a person's schedule of living or may be only a snack added to his regular meal pattern.

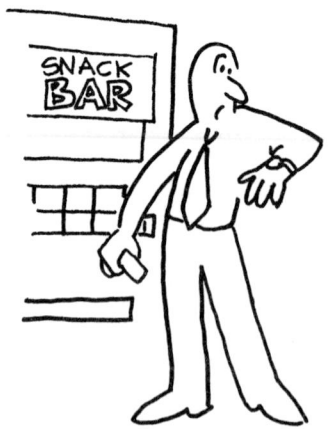

Fig. 4.6 Quick ready-to-eat food items purchased in vending machines may constitute a meal.

2. Meals eaten away from home comprise a number of major categories:
   (a) Lunches at school for children can be either in the school lunch program, packed-at-home lunches, or chance purchases at a nearby "spot."
   (b) Lunches for workers who live too far to return home to eat may choose

packed-at-home lunches, luncheonettes, "Blue Plate Specials," crowded cafeterias, snack bars, lunch-in-a-can, or the leisurely business-related lunch in a club.

(c) Social and professional eating away from home includes ladies' luncheons and the more elaborate dinners at night and on Sundays in which families relieve their feeling of boredom at home by eating out.

The food service industry is "Big Business" as indicated by the increasing numbers of cafeterias, catering services, in office or in industry food services, and fashionable restaurants often with gourmet-type specialities. In a nutshell, we need to learn how to eat out successfully which means:

- safe satisfying food
- clean pleasant food production and eating facilities
- good supply of nutrition which neither duplicates food eaten at home nor adds unnecessary calories to the diets of sedentary people
- servings adjusted to amount eaten avoiding quantities of plate waste

Some guidelines to eating-away-from-home include:

Select a place in which to eat by its general appearance of compliance with health and safe food production standards, a list of such establishments is available from city and state health departments:

(a) Usually those within city limits are checked more carefully and frequently than those in rural areas.

(b) "Back door" inspection or a "quick trip to the restroom" will establish an impression of management and compliance with regulations.

(c) Trained employees as evidenced by proper handling of equipment in setting and clearing tables in the dining area.

(d) Note seams and crevices in containers and in work or food service surfaces.

Select food on the bases of:

(a) the rest of the day's food consumption plan;

(b) a balanced assortment of nutrients, namely, a protein-rich source, one carbohydrate-rich food, not more than one high-fat food, if any, some fibrous, chewy or other low calorie but taste textured item;

(c) restrict total calorie intake in a single meal to not over one-half of the day's need, preferably only a fourth or a third should be consumed;

(d) restrain impulse ordering of excessive amounts or variety of foods to avoid overeating and/or plate waste.

Cautions to observe in eating out:

(a) Eat as near the regular mealtime as possible so food is more apt to be freshly prepared.

(b) Do not order seldom chosen items on the menu, e.g., chicken livers or oysters, unless these are being eaten by others; such foods may have been in storage for too long a period.

(c) Hot foods are more apt to be safe than cold ones, e.g., fried chicken in contrast to chicken salad.

(d) Certain foods should not be eaten in warm summer months unless their safety is assured, namely, custards, cream pies, puddings, and mixed sandwich fillings and salads containing eggs, ham, chicken, fish, or other cut up or ground precooked meats.

(e) If the majority of the daily meals are eaten out, a source of ascorbic acid and of B-complex vitamins may be needed to replace those lost in food preparation or not included in the meals.

Safe food

Bacteria multiply very rapidly under conditions favorable for their growth as can be seen in Fig 4.7. Each bacterium is multiplying at the rate of 500 times per 3 hours. At this fast rate: $500 \times 500 = 250,000$ bacteria in another 3 hours for every single one.

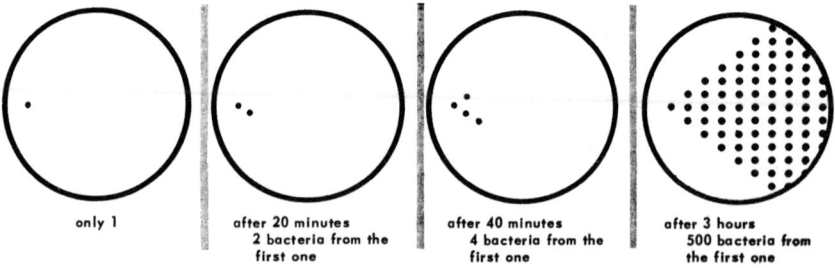

| only 1 | after 20 minutes
2 bacteria from the
first one | after 40 minutes
4 bacteria from the
first one | after 3 hours
500 bacteria from
the first one |

Fig. 4.7 The rate of bacterial growth is phenomenal.

Some factors which can affect bacterial growth are the:

1. degree of contamination — number of organisms present
2. temperature — keep cold food cold; keep hot food hot to reduce growth

3. food medium — acid and sugar foods do not support the growth rate that other foods do
4. duration — length of time involved is of major significance in total number of organisms in the food eaten.

The principle causes of foodborne disease outbreaks are:

1. failure to refrigerate perishable foods
2. food handling by diseased or contaminated employees
3. poor habits of personal hygiene of the employee or of the diner
4. failure to cook contaminated foods thoroughly
5. obtaining food from unsafe sources
6. failure to clean and disinfect kitchen utensils and equipment
7. poor food storage practices including keeping food on hand too long
8. use of the wrong equipment in food preparation such as utensils with seams, porous cutting boards, and others.

Since temperature is a crucial aspect of bacterial growth, to be familiar with significant temperatures is important. For quick reference, a diagram has been designed in Fig. 4.8 to direct attention to temperatures and to their relative relation to each other in helping to assure food safety.

Activities for Student Learning

1. You need to develop skill in the computation of the nutritive content of a recipe:
   The following recipe was prepared and served to 6 persons.

   MASHED POTATOES AU GRATIN: 6 Servings

Amount of Food	Ingredients	Weight in grams
4 med. sized	potatoes, peeled	544
1 tsp. salt	salt	6
2 Tbsp.	margarine	28
½ cup	hot milk	122
½ cup	grated cheddar cheese	56

   (a) Describe preparation and cooking procedure to give maximum retention of nutrients.
   (b) Calculate the nutrient content.
   (c) Analyze the influence of the items added to the potatoes on the calorie, protein, mineral and vitamin content of the recipe.

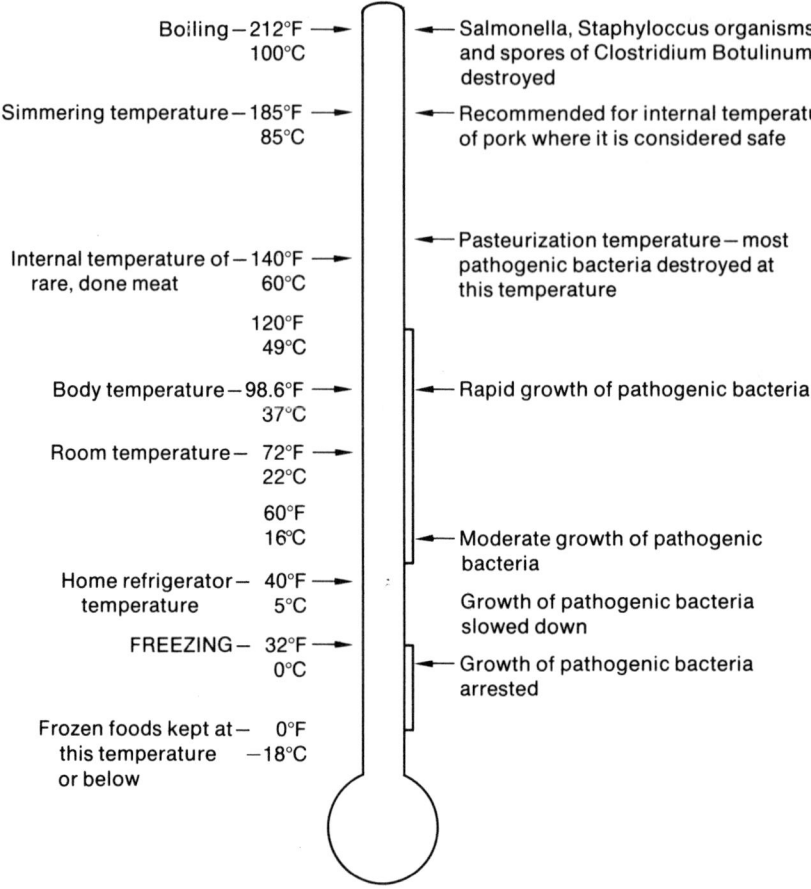

FAHRENHEIT AND CENTIGRADE SCALES

Fig. 4.8   Critical temperatures in food safety.

(d) Decide if this recipe would serve as an entree and make adjustments if required.

(e) Adjust the recipe for low, average, and high calorie dietaries.

2. You need to be able to develop recipes and establish their nutrient content to meet these specifications:

(a) A meat extender recipe which would be low cost and contain per serving at least 25% of the RDA for vitamin A.

(b) A bread, a serving of which would meet the requirements of an entree (have 15–20 g of protein per serving).

(c) Others to meet special dietary needs of you or of your family.

3. Acquire sterile agar plates, label, inoculate and incubate, to allow for bacterial growth. You may choose one of the suggested methods to serve as the inoculant:

   (a) sneezing
   (b) hair
   (c) piece of food dropped on the floor
   (d) touching with finger tips
   (e) touching with lips
   (f) saliva

4. You need to read the advertisements in one issue of a medical or dietetic journal and tabulate the dietary supplements and their nutrient contribution.

---

5. *Hot Tips:*

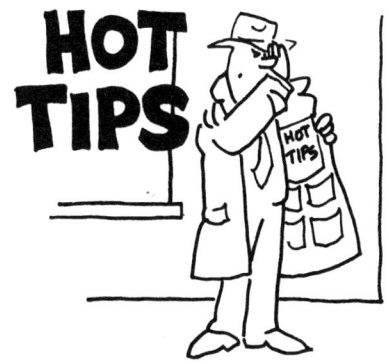

New Words:

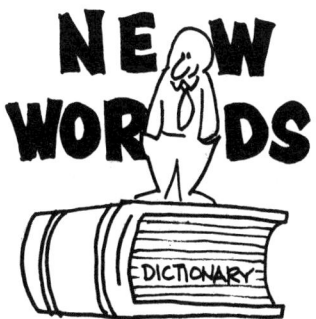

DIETARY ANALYSIS AS A TOOL IN EDUCATION AND RESEARCH

Objectives

1. To comprehend the significance of dietary analysis.
2. To realize that help in dietary improvement depends on understanding the food intake, acceptance, and ethnic values related to food of the person involved.
3. To be able to plan, conduct, and evaluate a dietary study of limited scope.

Dietary Analysis

Nutrition is the food we eat. Based on this premise, the use of dietary analysis to evaluate the food we eat and thereby the nutrient intake, becomes crucial in a study of human nutrition. To measure the relationship of dietary intake and of physiological response is one of the tasks confronting researchers in establishing the role of dietary practices to achieve optimal nutritional status. Data from one individual does not necessarily conform to the averages derived from groups of persons. Wide variations occur between individuals which make generalized statements only vaguely applicable to any one person. Dietary analysis is no exception; "one man's meat may be another's poison" has long been expressed as a phenomenon of individualism.

Obviously the best dietary analysis is the one in which all food to be eaten is measured or weighed and an aliquot taken for chemical analysis. For the aliquot, a given percentage of all foods eaten is analyzed which gives exact data on the dietary intake for that day or some other period of time.

Dietary analysis is the simplest method by which to assess the nutrient intake of an individual or of a group of people. Many problems are involved in order to make the analysis a quantitative measure of nutrient intake. An initial problem concerns the accuracy of determining the amount of food consumed. Weight, volumes, unit pieces, cans, packages, and additives become meaningful data to the dietary analyst. Another question involves the duration of time during which the sampling of dietary practices must be made to obtain a reliable indication of the food eaten by the person being studied. The study may concern only one meal like breakfast, although most studies are based on total daily consumption; the question is how many breakfasts or for how many days should amounts of food eaten be recorded? A researcher needs to decide whether the days should be consecutive, alternate, or inter-mittent; whether weekends, seasonal, or other specification.

Naturally, the problems are interrelated. The number of days re-quired for an accurate analysis depends on the variability of the diet it-self. Data on daily variations are limited but we could assume that during infancy and early childhood people eat regular consistent meals whereas, during adolescence behavioral variations cause similar aberrations in dietary practices.

Before any data are collected in a dietary study, the method of analysis needs to be designed. If food intake is to be analyzed chemically then aliquot samples must be collected. However, more often the "graphite-cellulose method of the armchair chemist" has been used and all data are computed from average values given in USDA Handbook No. 8 and other compilations of food composition. A list of books on food composition is included with references in Section 1. Such analyses listed in books are really an "edu-cated guess" at best. The assumption is that the accuracy is sufficient for the variability of the individual's dietary practices. After all, during meals, some food remains clinging to the dishes and is not consumed; to eat a "cup of beans" could mean to give or take a tablespoonful or two; even when portions are weighed, the plates are not rinsed in order to be able to eat the last remaining gram of

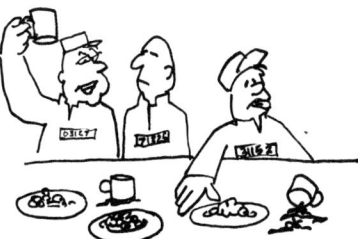

Fig. 4.9 Plate waste determines the amount of food eaten.

food. Chemical analysis of an aliquot of the food eaten is the preferred method but is very expensive and not always practical or even possible. Thus many dietary analyses are computational exercises which are adequate for education and routine medical and clinical uses.

Steps that can be followed in planning a dietary analysis include:

1. Select subject(s) appropriate for the problem and acquire demo-graphic data needed.
2. Determine size of sample required to establish purpose or test hypotheses.
3. Establish time period during which data on food consumption will be collected.
4. Record amounts of food consumed giving special attention to additives and snacks.

5. Tabulate foods into groups, preferably five groups to allow for a miscellaneous food group.
6. Calculate nutrient content by use of acceptable food composition tables.
7. Compute subtotals for food groups, total for period, and average the daily nutrient consumption or whatever combination is needed.
8. Calculate percentage deviation of intake from RDA; calculate percentage of nutrients derived from each food group.
9. Note significance of findings.
10. Compare results with those of other dietary studies.
11. Make recommendations by which to achieve change in the dietary habits of the person involved.

The National Nutrition Survey which started in 1969 was the first comprehensive survey to assess the nutritional status of the population of the United States. Final results from this survey were to present a reliable picture of the nutritional health status of people living in the lower income areas. Considerable delay occurred in release of data from the National Nutrition Survey; the survey itself has been discontinued as of 1970 when the director left to assume other responsibilities.

A summary of studies of *Dietary Adequacy and Nutritional Status in the United States* has been published in the Dairy Council Digest (1967). The summary represents a technic which can be used to establish the background for research projects involving a dietary survey.

Activities for Student Learning

1. You may want to read from some references which assess dietary study methods:

    Burke, B. S. The dietary history as a tool in research, *J. Amer. Dietet. Assoc.*, **23**, 1041 (1947).

    Carroll, M. E., *et al.* Group method of food inventory vs. individual study methods. II. Dietary history vs. seven-day record vs. 24-hr. recall, *J. Amer. Dietet. Assoc.*, **28**, 1146 (1952).

    Young, C. M., *et al.* A comparison of dietary study methods. I. Dietary history vs. seven-day record, *J. Amer. Dietet. Assoc.*, **28**, 124 (1952).

    Young, C. M., *et al.* A comparison of dietary study methods. II. Dietary history vs. seven-day record vs. 24-hr. recall, *J. Amer. Dietet. Assoc.*, **28**, 218 (1952).

Young, C. M., *et al.* Cooperative nutritional status studies in the North-east region. III. Contributions to dietary methodology studies, *Agr. Exp. Sta. Bull.*, No. 469. Amherst, Mass.: University of Massachusetts, 1952.

Young, C. M., *et al.* Methodology for dietary studies in epidemiological surveys. II. Strengths and weaknesses of existing methods. *Amer. J. Public Health*, **50**, 803 (1960).

2. Locate, read, and report to your classmates information from recent publications on the current National Nutrition Survey (1969–70).
3. You and your classmates could design and role play a hypothetical dietary study. Consider the human relation elements involved, the choice of the different instruments for use and the various procedures in collecting and evaluating the dietary information. (Be able to give concrete instructions to a participant in such a study.)
4. You may wish to view a film on a dietary survey such as the one, *Nutrition in Texas*. Texas State Dept. Health, Austin, Texas 78711.

References and Suggested Readings

Baker, H., Frank, O., Feingold, S., Christakis, G., and Ziffer, H. Vitamins total cholesteral and triglycerides in 642 New York City school children, *Amer. J. Clin. Nutr.*, **20**, 850 (1967).

Brin, M., Dibble, M. V., Peel, A., McMullen, E., Bourquin, A., and Chen, N. Some preliminary findings on the nutritional status of the aged in Onodaga, Canada, *Amer. J. Clin. Nutr.*, **17**, 240 (1965).

Dierks, E. C., and Morse, L. M. Some preliminary findings in junior high school children in Syracuse and Onodaga County, New York, *J. Amer. Dietet. Assoc.*, **47**, 292 (1965).

Dietary adequacy and nutritional status in the U.S., National Dairy Council Digest, 1967.

Dietary levels of households in the United States, Spring 1965, USDA ARS 62-17 (January 1968).

Elwood, P. C., and Waters, W. E. The vital distinction, *Nutr. Today*, **4**, 14 (1969).

Eppright, E. W., Fox, H. M., Fryer, B. A., Lamkin, G. H., and Vivian, V. M. Eating behavior of preschool children, *J. Nutr. Educ.*, **1**, 16 (1969).

Family food plans and food costs, Rev. 1964, CA 62-19 USDA ARS, Hyattsville, Md. (1969).

Forums in focus, *Food Tech.*, **24**, 269 (1970).

Goddard, J. L. Incident at Selby Junior High, *Nutr. Today*, **2**, 2 (1967).

Goldsmith, G. A. The new dietary allowances, *Nutr. Today*, **3**: 4, 16 (1968).

Hampton, M. C., Huenemann, R. L., Shapiro, L. R., and Mitchell, B. W. Calorie and nutrient intakes of teenagers, *J. Amer. Dietet. Assoc.*, **50**, 385 (1967).

Hodges, R. E., and Krehl, W. A. Nutritional status of teenagers in Iowa, *Amer. J. Clin. Nutr.*, **17**, 200 (1965).

Jerome, N. W., and Pringle, D. J. Sociocultural factors and food habits of in-migrant families, *Amer. Dietet. Assoc.* meeting (August 18, 1967).

LeBovit, C. J. The food of older persons living at home, *J. Amer. Dietet. Assoc.*, **46**, 285 (1965).

Lindsay, D. R. Food safety, *FDA Papers*, **4**, 4 (1970).

Lund, L. A. Study of children's food consumption behavior, *Amer. Home Eco. Assoc.* meeting (June 27, 1967).

Parrish, J. B. Implications of changing food habits for nutrition educators, *J. Nutr. Educ.*, **2**: 4, 140 (1971).

Recommended Dietary Allowances, 7th ed. Washington, D.C.: National Academy of Sciences, 1968.

Sandstead, H. H., Carter, J. P., and Darby, W. J. How to diagnose nutritional disorders in daily practice, *Nutr. Today*, **4**, 20 (1969).

Schaefer, A. E. Are we well fed? The search for the answer, *Nutr. Today*, **4**, 2 (1969).

INVENTORY OF KNOWLEDGE

Part I

Some of these statements are true and some are false. Indicate your reaction by a circle around T or F for each statement:

T   F   1. Food guides are designed to aid in planning well-balanced meals.

T   F   2. Nutrition can be related to the behavioral and social sciences.

T   F   3. A popular concept is that all good food is fattening.

T   F   4. Criticism and nagging will result in a person's development of recommended food habits.

T   F   5. Regularity of eating is essential for adequate nutrient intake.

T   F   6. Children should be permitted to make food choices, e.g., the child can choose whether to drink sweet milk or chocolate milk, either hot or cold.

T   F   7. The wise mother can add needed nutrients to the food that her family will consume.

T   F   8. Low-cost foods usually are less nutritious than more expensive ones.

T   F   9. Serving milk with peanut butter and crackers makes the vegetable protein more useful to the body.

T   F   10. Dried fruits are valuable sources of ascorbic acid.

T   F   11. The best-liked foods in the United States are beef, potatoes, bread, and desserts.

T   F   12. Increased length of cooking time when preparing vegetables may be more destructive than an increased temperature with short time.

T F   13. Dietary supplements are generally unwarranted in the diets of families in the United States in most instances.

Part II   Multiple Choice

Select the best choice(s) to answer the following questions or complete the statement and circle your selection:

14. Milk is the main source of calcium in the American diet; adequate substitutes for an 8 oz serving of milk are:
    (a) $1\frac{1}{4}$ oz cheddar cheese
    (b) $\frac{1}{2}$ C creamed cottage cheese
    (c) 4 oz ice cream
    (d) $\frac{1}{2}$ C pudding
    (e) all of the above

15. Four or more servings from the fruit and vegetable group are needed daily. Which of the following suggestions would be the best choice for a normal adult?
    (a) broccoli, orange juice, squash, potato
    (b) spinach, pear nectar, carrots, corn
    (c) onions, tomato juice, cauliflower, lettuce
    (d) green beans, orange juice, tomato, grapefruit
    (e) celery, pineapple, juice, pear, banana

16. Water soluble nutrients *can be lost* during the preparation of foods by many methods which may include:
    (a) using a minimum amount of cooking water
    (b) vaporization in the steam during cooking
    (c) using the vegetable liquor in sauces or gravies
    (d) discarding water in which vegetables were soaked
    (e) using a pan with a fitted lid for cooking that is related to the burner size

17. Certain vitamins are readily destroyed by heat, examples of these are:
    (a) thiamine and vitamin A
    (b) ascorbic acid and thiamine
    (c) vitamin A and ascorbic acid
    (d) riboflavin and ascorbic acid
    (e) thiamine and niacin

18. One would expect more nutrients to be preserved in which of the following foods?
    (a) toasted bread
    (b) browned rolls
    (c) green beans cooked with soda
    (d) loaf of bread
    (e) celery pieces stored in jar of water

19. The temperature range which is most favorable for growth of pathogenic bacteria is:
    (a) 0–32°F
    (b) 34–40°F
    (c) 40–140°F
    (d) 140–185°F
    (e) 185–212°F

20. The temperature range which retards bacterial growth and is used only for temporary food storage in the refrigerator is:
    (a) 0–32°F
    (b) 34–40°F
    (c) 40–140°F
    (d) 140–185°F
    (e) 185–212°F

5

The Body's Need for Nutrients: Dietary Supply

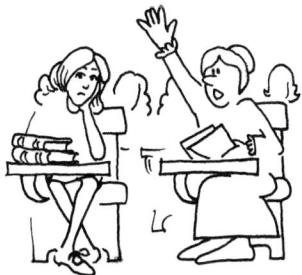

Fig. 5.1 "I've studied about carbohydrates, fats, and protein since the third grade—do I have to do it again?"

The first and most basic need of the body is for energy. The term, energy comes from the word *energos* meaning "active": *en* (in) and *ergon* (work). In physics, work is defined as the product of weight times distance, for example, the amount of work required to move a liter (1 kg) of blood through 5 meters of blood vessels or a 100 pound body a distance of two city blocks. Movement as defined in work is often referred to as *kinetic energy* which is illustrated by the force of any moving object such as fluidity of blood, an avalanche of water or wind flying a kite. Basically the energy of life is kinetic energy involved in the multiple movement of fluids and chemical exchanges included in the term metabolism.

Another type is potential energy, the energy inherent in food. The potential energy value of food is bound in the chemical bonds of the elements in three major or macronutrients; carbohydrates, fats, and proteins. This energy can be released only by complex enzyme systems which contain vitamins and mineral elements. The interrelated metabolic behavior of the major nutrients clearly implies that dietary

97

manipulation in the ratio of carbohydrates, fats, and proteins may have far-reaching effects upon the metabolism and function of the body.

FOOD AS A SOURCE OF ENERGY

Objectives

1. To recognize the processes of photosynthesis as the origin of food for human nutrition and that the chemical composition determines the potential energy value.
2. To identify the sequence in which organic compounds are changed from those in food to nutrients in the blood.
3. To be able to compute the potential energy value of a given amount of a food and dietaries for family groups of different age, activity, and health.

Production of Potential Energy in Food

All of the energy on earth originates from the sun. Chlorophyll in plant cells packages the energy into carbohydrate molecules; thus plants serve as food for animals (herbivora) which in turn may be eaten by other animals (carnivora). Some animals including man consume food from both plants and animals (omnivora).

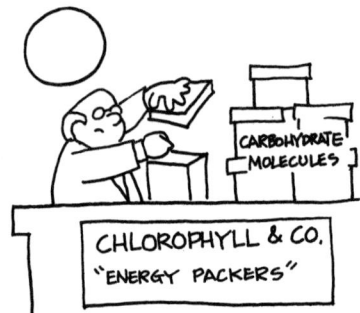

Fig. 5.2   Plant cells package energy into carbohydrate molecules.

Carbohydrates

What are Carbohydrates?

Carbohydrates are the preferred fuel for use by the body and represent the largest single component of most diets other than water. Carbohydrates were one of the first nutrients to be chemically identified; the ratio of hydrogen to oxygen is $2:1$, the same ratio as found in water — hence the term carbohydrate.

In the process of metabolism, carbon is oxidized to carbon dioxide and hydrogen to water, thereby releasing energy characteristic of this type of molecule:

$$C_6H_{12}O_6 + 6O_2 \longrightarrow 6CO_2 + 6H_2O + energy$$

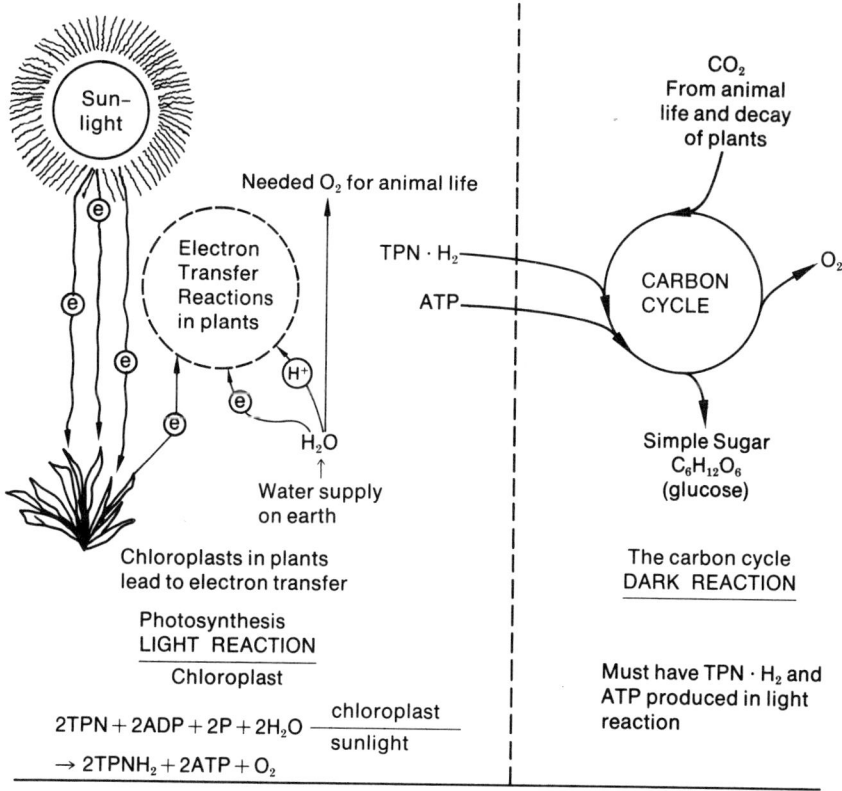

Basic formula for the two phases of photosynthesis:

$$6CO_2 + 12H_2O \longrightarrow C_6H_{12}O_6 + 6O_2 + 6H_2O$$

Terms used:

ⓔ	electron transfer reactions
TPN · H$_2$	Triphosphopyridine Nucleotide plus two molecules of hydrogen
ATP	Adenosine triphosphate: ⎡adenosine⎤—Ⓟ—Ⓟ—Ⓟ
	a complex organic molecule that is the source for energy

Fig. 5.3 Schema for production of energy.

The simplest structural unit of carbohydrate is the monosaccharide. Most monosaccharides in foods are hexoses since they are composed of a six-carbon-unit to which hydrogen and oxygen atoms are attached both as hydrogen (H^+) and as hydroxyl (OH^-) groups. The three monosaccharides in food released by digestive processes and of importance in nutrition are glucose, fructose, and galactose which contain the same number and kinds of atoms — six carbon atoms, twelve hydrogen atoms,

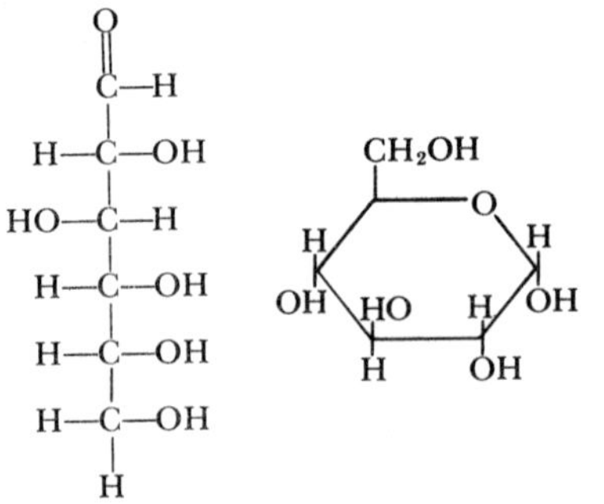

$C_6H_{12}O_6$

Fig. 5.4 Two methods to illustrate the structure of glucose.

and six oxygen atoms, as shown in Fig. 5.4. These are spacially arranged around the chain of carbon atoms or its cyclic configuration. These different arrangements of atoms account for the variation in sweetening power, solubility, and other properties of the different monosaccharides.

Two molecules of monosaccharides are combined to form a disaccharide with the release of one molecule of water. Thus glucose units are joined together to produce a larger molecule, in this case, the double sugar maltose. This process is called dehydration synthesis. The reverse process, whereby maltose is broken down by the chemical addition of water between two units, is called hydrolysis. Such processes, dehydration synthesis and hydrolysis occur in the construction and degradation of all major carbohydrate macromolecules (large molecules built by repeating smaller units) in the living cell.

$$C_6H_{12}O_6 + C_6H_{12}O_6 \longrightarrow C_{12}H_{22}O_{11} + H_2O$$
Monosaccharide Monosaccharide   Disaccharide   Water

Glucose, fructose, and galactose are three monosaccharides that are released from food during digestive processes and absorbed by the portal vein to be transported to the liver. From the liver, only glucose is released for circulation into the blood. Glucose, sometimes referred to as dextrose or grape sugar is readily used by most organisms as a source of energy. The disaccharides commonly found in foods are sucrose, lactose, and maltose. The most familiar in household use is sucrose, known as cane or beet sugar.

The third group of carbohydrates, the polysaccharides—starches, dextrins, glycogen, and celluloses, are complex molecules of hundreds of units of the monosaccharide, glucose. The cellulose and starch molecules can be degradated stepwise to produce simpler starches, then to the disaccharide maltose, and finally to glucose. This process is used to

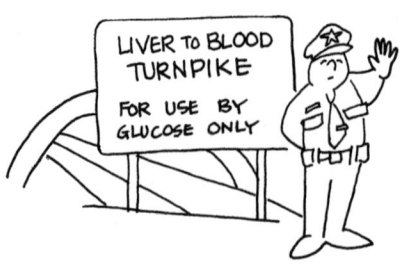

Fig. 5.5 The liver releases only glucose to the blood.

produce corn syrup and cornsugar (glucose) from cornstarch. Corn syrup, which is a mixture of dextrins, maltose and glucose, and glucose are about half as sweet as sucrose. Starch is the main energy storage reserve for most plants and one of the most important energy sources for man. Human liver and muscles store limited amounts of carbohydrate in the form of glycogen, sometimes called animal starch. In a well-fed adult person the glycogen content of the liver may be 100–200 g or just less than ½ lb in a 3–4 lb liver. The glycogen content of beef or pork liver constitutes about 2–6% of its raw weight. This amount of glycogen is significant in planning carbohydrate controlled diets. In muscles, the glycogen concentration is transitory and negligible in amount and quickly utilized in energy metabolism.

Cellulose is the most abundant carbohydrate in nature. These complex carbohydrate molecules, polysaccharides, have no fixed size and may contain up to 10,000 glucose units. Cellulose can be used by ruminating animals whose multiple stomachs contain certain single cell organisms which inhabit the rumen and degradate the complex molecules forming not only utilizable carbohydrates but also high concentrations of proteins (30–70% of dry weight residues).

The use of cellulose as utilizable food for people was developed by Hitler's scientific organization prior to World War II. He used soft wood pulp as sources of cellulose to be degradated by strong acids into maltose- and glucose-rich syrups termed "ersatz zucher." Other cellulose wastes were used to grow torula-type yeasts which produced in a few days, tons of high protein residues of high biological value. Hungry people ate these products, but today no evidence exists of their continued use as food for people who are in less desperate situations and have more abundant food supplies.

Activities for Student Learning

1. You will want to read a chapter on carbohydrates in some selected book (or ones listed in Section 1) to identify the functions performed by carbohydrate in the body.
2. Can you enumerate the factors which affect the digestion and absorption of carbohydrates?
3. You may plot a bar graph showing the percentage of carbohydrate for the following foods: whole grain bread, molasses, cornflakes, cooked beans, oranges, ground beef, and table sugar.
4. When you need to plan a reducing diet, which carbohydrate foods should you include and which should you omit? What is the rationale for such decisions?

5. You need to calculate the carbohydrate content of several "made" desserts and note ingredients which are the chief contributors of sugars and starches.

6. You will want to survey local food processors and compute the composition of some standard commercial formulas for foods such as pastries, ice creams, etc. and identify their sugar, starch, and fat contents.

7. Did you remember to fill in the following?

Hot Tips:

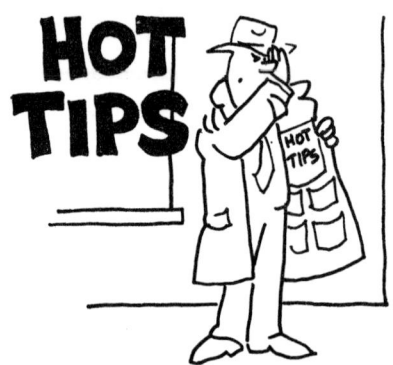

New Words:

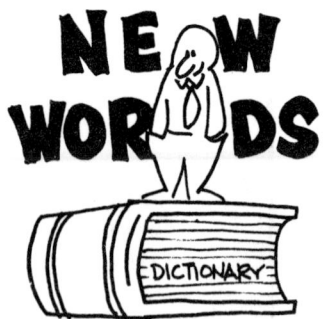

Lipids and Fats

The broad classification of lipids embraces all substances extractable from biological materials with the usual fat solvents (ether, acetone, chloroform, alcohol, etc.) and includes the fat soluble vitamins, fats, and compounds of metabolic importance such as phospholipids, glycolipids, cholesterol, and others.

What are fats? All fats are insoluble in water; other physical and chemical properties vary with the types, proportions, and arrangement of fatty acids in the molecule. The fat macromolecules, like those of carbohydrates, are composed of carbon, hydrogen, and oxygen, yet fats contain over twice the energy value of carbohydrates (nine calories per gram for fats and four calories per gram for carbohydrates). The difference in energy value lies in the proportion of oxidizable elements

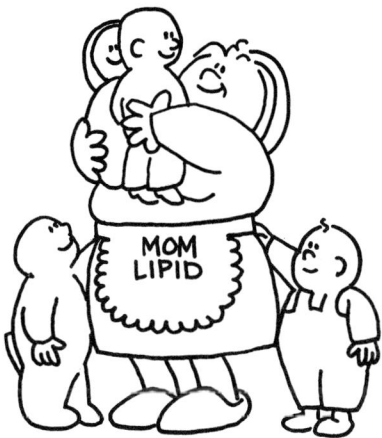

Fig. 5.6 A lipid releases fatty acids and embraces many substances.

in the molecule. Fats contain a much higher ratio of carbon and hydrogen in the molecule than of oxygen; i.e., less intramolecular oxidation than in carbohydrates. A molecule of fat contains three fatty acids and glycerol, which is a type of alcohol. These are joined together as an ester, a particular type of chemical combination of bonds between certain types of atoms. Because of this structural composition, fats are called triglycerides with structures formed as follows:

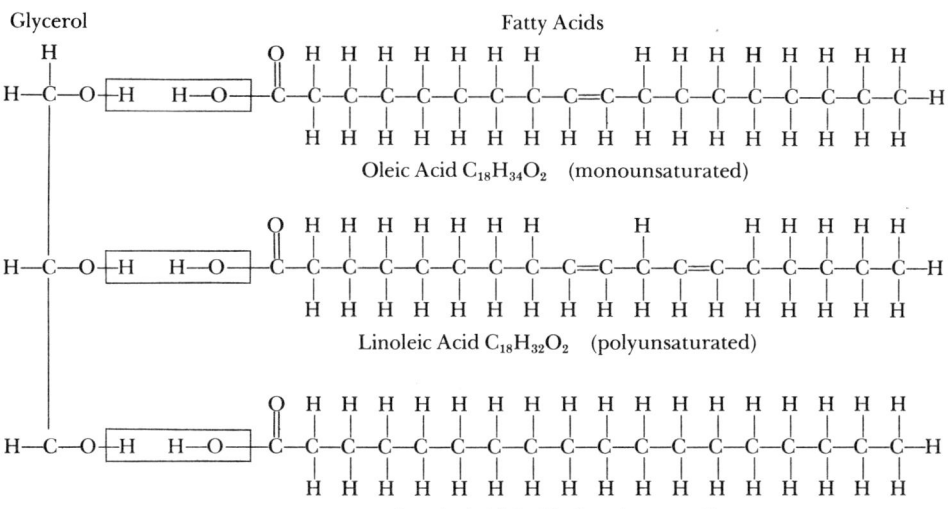

When a fat molecule is formed, the hydrogen atom of glycerol combines with the hydroxyl radical of the fatty acid to link the glycerol to each of the three fatty acids. Water (HOH) is formed as a by-product. Thus a triglyceride and three molecules of metabolic water are produced. The fatty acids which form a triglyceride may be three molecules of the same fatty acid, of different fatty acids or of any combination. Furthermore, the position on the glycerol occupied by each fatty acid makes a difference. When only one or two molecules of fatty acids are added, the product is a mono- or diglyceride; such compounds are used as emulsifying agents in food processing.

Fatty acids classified according to the number of carbons in the straight chain linkage would have these dimensions:

Short chain — C_4, C_6 and sometimes C_8
Medium chain — C_8, C_{10}, C_{12}, C_{14}
Long chain — C_{16}, C_{18}, C_{20}, and longer

Fats composed of shorter chain fatty acids have lower melting points (liquid at room temperatures of 70–72°F); conversely, those with longer chain acids have higher melting points. The properties of fats are dependent both on the length of the chain and on the "degree of saturation" of fatty acids. A carbon atom may have four other atoms bonded to it; in a saturated fatty acid, the bonds are saturated or filled to capacity with hydrogen. Note the formula given for stearic acid as compared to oleic and linoleic acids. When the bonds of the carbon atoms are not connected to other elements, two bonds connect two carbon atoms which is referred to as a double bond (note the formula for oleic acid); thus the fatty acid is said to be unsaturated. If only one double bond is present, the fatty acid is called monounsaturated; whereas the presence of two or more double bonds is termed polyunsaturated (note the formula for linoleic acid).

Fats that are solid at room temperature are composed of saturated fatty acids, which is characteristic of most fats of animal origin; those liquid at room temperature have a higher percentage of unsaturated fatty acids. For example, large amounts of saturated stearic acid are found in suet, the more unsaturated oleic acid occurs in olive oil, and the polyunsaturated linoleic acid occurs in oils from corn, cottonseed, and soybean.

All seed oils are liquid at room temperature and contain a high proportion of unsaturated and polyunsaturated fatty acids. Fats from each species of animals and plants are distinctive; usually fat from herbivora has more saturated fatty acids than that from sea animals, and fat from four-legged animals is more saturated than that from two-legged ones (poultry), such as beef versus chicken. Oils extracted from seeds are the highest in polyunsaturated fatty acids of all natural fats, whereas oils from fruits may contain up to 90% of the monounsaturated fatty acid, oleic acid (found in olive and coconut oils). The unsaturated fatty acids usually are C_{18} and C_{20} acids.

Double bonds in fatty acids represent centers of chemical activity; when oxidation occurs at the double bond, the change in the fat is identified as rancidity. The ease with which oils become rancid has been a detriment to their use in food. In the 1920s a process was developed that added hydrogen at the double bond and changed an oil into a fat which was solid at room temperature. In fact, the "hardness" of the fat at a given temperature can be controlled by the degree to which the polyunsaturated fatty acids have been changed to monounsaturated and finally to saturated fatty acids. For example:

$$C_{18}H_{32}O_2 \xrightarrow{+H_2} C_{18}H_{34}O_2 \xrightarrow{+H_2} C_{18}H_{36}O_2$$

Linoleic	Oleic	Stearic
Dominant in	Dominant in	Dominant in
seed oils	oleomargarine	animal fats such
		as tallow

Medium chain triglycerides (MCT) have recently become prominent in research and are being provided by a manufacturing company as a special source of fat. These triglycerides contain octanoic and decanoic acids, C_8 and C_{10} fatty acids, respectively. These triglycerides are digested and absorbed differently from triglycerides composed of long chain fatty acids which comprise about 98% of most dietary fats. Medium chain triglycerides require less enzymes and bile acids for digestion than conventional food fat. They are transported directly by the portal circulation, while regular food fat requires the more complex intestinal micellar formation and chylomicron transport system of the lymph. The usual result is markedly increased availability of fat calories. The MCT may be useful in nutritional management of persons with impaired digestion or malabsorption of fats such as occurs in steatorrhea, neonatal hepatitis, or cirrhosis. The unique MCT oil is a trademark licensed from Dow Chemical Company and is on the market for use in special dietary products prescribed by doctors and sold in pharmacies.

Even though the body uses fat mainly as fuel, it is essential for health and is indispensable in the diet. However, any attempt to utilize appreciable quantities of fat without concomitant degradation of an adequate amount of carbohydrate can lead to ketosis, hypercholesterolemia, hyperlipemia, or fatty liver.

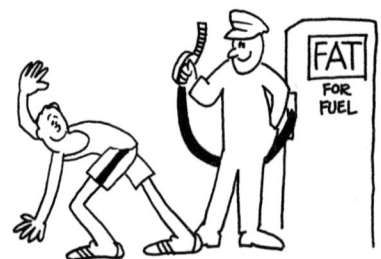

Fig. 5.7 The body uses fat mainly as fuel.

The current concern about the role of dietary fats in cardiovascular disasters, has directed attention to the ratio of polyunsaturated to saturated fatty acids and to the ratio of short chain to medium to long chain fatty acids. Early research indicated that vegetable oils were effective in reducing serum cholesterol. A standard recommendation found in many diet manuals states specific polyunsaturated/saturated (P/S) ratio of 2:1.

Activities for Student Learning

1. You need to read about lipids and fats in a suitable reference.
2. You should determine the physical characteristics (odor, texture, color, taste) of stearic, linoleic, and oleic fatty acids; also of margarine, lard, shortening, olive oil, cod liver oil, corn oil, chicken fat, lamb fat, etc. You need to compare the texture to the amount of saturated fatty acids present.
3. Prepare a graph showing the percentage of total fat in descending order for the following: lard, butter, margarine, bacon, potato chips, cottonseed oil, avocado, chocolate bar, plain cake, white enriched bread, ground hamburger meat, and mayonnaise.
4. Could you plan a diet with the polyunsaturated/saturated (P/S) ratio recommended for healthful living?

Protein as a Source of Energy

What Is the Role of Protein as a Source of Energy?

Proteins are relatively large molecules composed of amino acids linked together through the amine group ($-NH_2$) of one molecule and the carboxyl ($-COOH$) group of another.

$$R-\underset{\underset{NH_2}{|}}{\overset{\overset{H}{|}}{C}}-COOH$$

Any alpha amino acid where R represents any number of different radicals. Alpha refers to the first carbon following the carboxyl group ($-COOH$).

The $-NH_2^-$ group of any amino acid can combine with the $-COOH^+$ group of another, forming a spiral shaped linkage of hundreds of amino acids to synthesize a single protein molecule. This buildup of the specified sequence of amino acid molecules attached by peptide linkage to form a protein molecule is termed protein synthesis. This synthesis occurs in a stepwise progress of two amino acids combining to form a dipeptide:

$$H-\underset{\underset{NH_2}{|}}{\overset{\overset{H}{|}}{C}}-COOH + \underset{\underset{H}{|}}{\overset{\overset{H}{|}}{N}}\!\!-\!\!\underset{\underset{COOH}{|}}{\overset{\overset{H}{|}}{C}}-CH_3 \quad \underset{\text{hydrolysis}}{\overset{\text{synthesis}}{\rightleftharpoons}} \quad H-\underset{\underset{NH_2}{|}}{\overset{\overset{H}{|}}{C}}\!\!-\!\!\overset{\overset{O}{\|}}{C}-\underset{}{\overset{\overset{H}{|}}{N}}-\underset{\underset{COOH}{|}}{\overset{\overset{H}{|}}{C}}-CH_2 + H_2O$$

Amino Acid + Amino Acid   Dipeptide
e.g., glycine e.g., alanine

After dipeptide formation another amino acid can be added to form a tripeptide and so on until polypeptides and eventually protein molecules have been synthesized. These are reversible reactions and can proceed for synthesis of a protein molecule or for degradation of the protein as occurs during digestion.

Some 20 amino acids have been identified in natural protein molecules ranging from glycine, the smallest and simplest amino acid, to complex ones such as tryptophan. These amino acids are released from protein molecules by the process of hydrolysis catalyzed by digestive enzymes. Thus dietary proteins furnish amino acids which can be used not only as building material for body tissue, enzymes, and hormones but also can be used as a source of energy. If the total energy intake is too low, additional amino acids must be deaminated and the carbon-hydrogen skeleton can be oxidized to yield energy. In this way protein is used to meet the first demand of the body which is the requirement for energy. If the energy intake is adequate but protein intake is higher than required, the extra amino acids can be used to supply energy or to form fat to be stored in adipose tissue.

The oxidation of amino acids for energy requires that the amino acid first loses its amino group, leaving the carbon-hydrogen skeleton for oxidation or for fat synthesis. The amino group is removed by processes described as transamination or deamination. Transamination involves the production of other nitrogenous compounds such as those amino acids that can be synthesized in the body. Deamination removes the amino group which is then synthesized into urea which constitutes the main nitrogenous product excreted in the urine.

Activities for Student Learning

1. Please design or diagram the destiny of the protein content of a diet that is deficient in meeting the energy expenditure of a child.

2. Explain the role of protein as a source of energy in high protein reducing diets.
3. Plan a typical high protein and low calorie regimen for weight reduction, e.g., 100–150 g of protein in a 1200 calorie diet; compute the grams of protein, carbohydrate, and fat of the foods to be used as well as the cost of the food in the food groups to prepare this diet.

DIGESTIBILITY OF FOODS

Objectives

1. To be able to trace food during its passage through the digestive tract, identifying what happens in the bolus and chyme stages of digestion.
2. To distinguish how the composition of food and its physical properties affect its digestibility.

The Release of Nutrients by the Digestive System of Man

Food which is the recognized sole source of nutrients must undergo many changes before the nutrients are made available to the cells for utilization. The four basic steps in the release and utilization of nutrients are:

1. ingestion or taking food into the body,
2. digestion or release of nutrients from the food,
3. absorption or the process in which the end products of digestion pass through the wall of the gastrointestinal tract, and
4. transport of the nutrients by the blood to all body cells for ultimate utilization.

Each animal has a unique digestive system adapted to its dietary habits which includes what it eats, how much is ingested at a time, and consequently, the frequency of eating. An outline of man's organs for digestion and the general activity in each is given in Table 5.1.

Digestion of Food

As shown in the diagrams, Tables 5.2, 5.3, and 5.4, the end products of digestion are monosaccharides, fatty acids and glycerol, and amino acids. Digestion is characterized by:

1. A physical change occurs in the ingested food by a change from the

Table 5.1 The digestive system of man.

Organ	Changes Resulting from Digestive Process
Mouth:	
1. breakdown of food by tongue and cheek muscles and teeth	
2. food moistened by alkaline saliva (pH 6.4–7.3)	starch + salivary amylase → maltose
3. mucin, a glycoprotein, binds food into ball or bolus to be swallowed	
Stomach:	
1. elastic muscular pouch for storage	starch digestion continues until bolus is acid
2. circular and longitudinal muscles churn and mix food	movement separates food into smaller particles referred to
3. lining contains millions of tiny gastric glands	as chyme, a milky paste-like blend of food and fluids
4. hydrochloric acid (HCl) provides pH 1.5–4 for pepsin; denatures protein	protein + HCl + pepsin → proteoses, peptones, polypeptides
5. very limited amount of lipase	fat (emulsified only) + lipase → fatty acids + glycerol
Small Intestines:	
1. duodenum — first section of small intestines	fat saponified by bile, then pancreatic lipase → fatty acids
— bile duct supplies bile	and glycerol
— pancreatic juice supplies lipase, trypsinogen, chymotrypsin, amylase, carboxypolypeptidase	protein + trypsin → amino acids starch + amylase → maltose sucrose + sucrase → glucose + fructose
2. intestinal glands secrete monosaccharidases	maltose + maltase → glucose
3. small intestine primarily area for absorption of nutrients	lactose + lactase → glucose + galactose peptides + erepsin → amino acids
Large Intestine:	
1. large, lax tube	no digestion
2. bacteria produce some vitamins, gases and other compounds	water absorption
Colon and Anus: Waste (feces) eliminated, contains:	
1. indigestible cellulose	
2. nondigested portions of nutrients 8% protein 4% fat 2% CHO	
3. excreted mucus and enzymes from digestion	
4. degraded body cells	

Table 5.2   Physiological breakdown of carbohydrates from food.

Process	Changes Achieved		

Ingestion

Monosaccharides	Disaccharides	Polysaccharides	
		Starches	Celluloses
	Sucrose	Dextrins	Alphacel
	Maltose	Glycogen	Amylopectin
	Lactose		
	Gastric acidity		
	Intestinal	Salivary	
	Sucrase	Intestinal	
	Maltase	Amylase	
	Lactase	Maltase	

Absorption   Monosaccharides

$\downarrow$

Liver   Glycogen

$\downarrow$

Circulation   Glucose

$\downarrow$

Metabolism   Hexose phosphate

$\downarrow$

Energy $\leftarrow$ Glycogen $\leftrightarrow$ Fat synthesis

$\updownarrow$

Fat deposit

Excretion $CO_2 + H_2O$ Feces

solid to a semifluid form which is called chyme, this results from mechanical action in the mouth and stomach.

2. Peristaltic movements, caused by longitudinal and circular muscles, result in a coordinated wavelike contraction followed by relaxed rhythmic segmentation. These regular contractions of muscles cause fragmentation of the food mass. Also, such movements may cause the gastrointestinal contents to progress at different rates; either with normal motility, hypomotility which can be so slow as to cause constipation, or hypermotility such as occurs in diarrhea.

3. Chemical changes occur in which large molecules are changed to smaller ones, thereby increasing the solubility of nutrients.

These end products of digestion have three features in common:

1. they are small molecules that can pass through the cell membranes of the intestinal mucosa to be used by the body,

Table 5.3 Changes that fat from food undergoes during digestion, absorption, and metabolic processes to release energy and form body lipids.

Process	Changes Achieved
Ingestion ⟶	Dietary fats (triglycerides) and other lipids
Digestion ⟶	Gastric lipase Bile for saponification of fat Pancreatic lipase
Absorption ⟶	Lacteal of lymph → general circulation Long-chain fatty acids Glycerides Other lipids and Portal vein → Liver → general circulation Short-chain fatty acids Glycerol
Circulation ⟶	Free fatty acids Triglycerides Neutral fat Other lipids
Metabolism ⟶	Energy for muscular function Oxidation Lipid synthesis to form (1) Triglycerides → subcutaneous fat → visceral fat → organ fat (2) Other lipids ⟶ cholesterol ⟶ phospholipids Energy ↓
Excretion ⟶	$CO_2 + H_2O$

2. they are all sources of energy, or
3. they can be used to rebuild body tissues.

Mucosal cells line the small intestinal wall through which these small molecules must pass. The surface area of the intestinal wall is increased by villi, these are small projections from the wall, each of which contains

Table 5.4 Sequence of compounds involved in the change from protein food to amino acids and the synthesis of body protein.

Process	Changes Achieved
Ingestion $\longrightarrow$	Dietary Protein
Digestion $\longrightarrow$	Gastric proteinase (pepsin) Pancreatic proteinase (trypsin) Intestinal proteinase (erepsin)
Absorption $\longrightarrow$	Amino acids
Circulation $\longrightarrow$	Amino acids (soluble proteins)
Metabolism $\longrightarrow$	Synthesis Transamination Deamination $\quad NH_2 \to$ urea $\longrightarrow$ urine $\quad$ C—H skeleton $\to$ fat synthesis $\qquad\qquad\qquad\downarrow$ $\qquad\qquad$ Energy $\qquad\qquad\quad\downarrow$
Excretion $\longrightarrow$	$\qquad\qquad CO_2 + H_2O \qquad$ urine

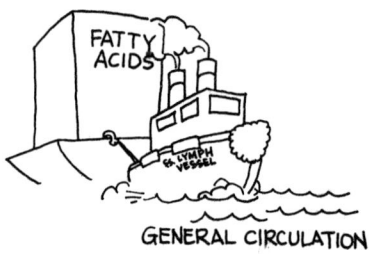

GENERAL CIRCULATION

Fig. 5.8 Absorption of fatty acids.

capillaries and a lacteal lymph vessel. Absorption in general depends upon the:

1. molecular size of the nutrients,
2. concentration of molecules on each side or the gradient on either side of a membrane such as the intestinal mucosa,
3. preferential selection of the intestinal mucosal membrane.

Simple sugars, amino acids, some fatty acids and glycerol, mineral and vitamins pass through the cells of the villi and enter the blood capillaries. Some products of fat digestion pass through the cells of the villi but enter the lymph lacteals instead of the blood capillaries. Eventually the lymph vessels bring the fat products into the general circulation.

Digestive enzymes have certain properties which help to explain digestive functions. Enzymes are:

(a) specific in action to cause the chemical change which each produces; at no time can one substitute for another in any area,

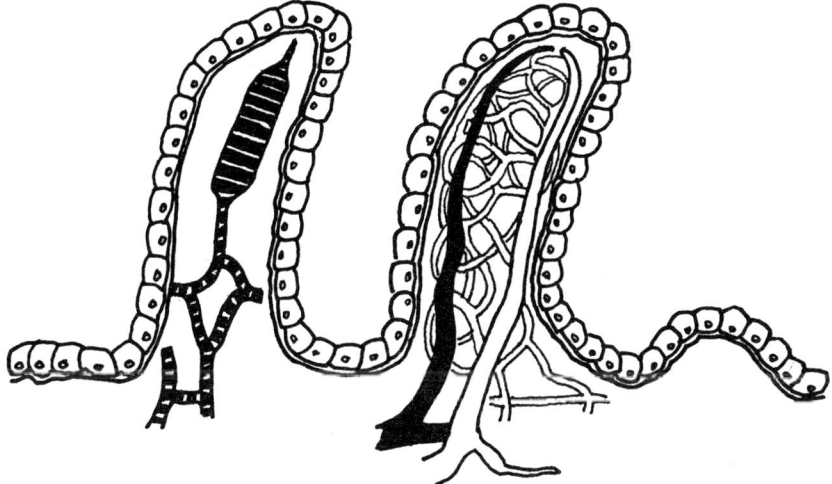

Fig. 5.9 Villi in the intestinal mucosa.

(b) very selective of the environmental conditions under which they will perform, the temperature range is narrow, the acidity specific, and often other ions or compounds need to be present,

(c) catalytic in action; the enzymes do not appear in the final product, and

(d) unstable and have to be produced continually to supply the body's needs.

Enzymes are named by a systematic nomenclature which shows the place of action and the substance acted upon. The suffix -ase means enzyme; e.g., salivary amylase or gastric proteinase. Proteinases are secreted in inactive forms to prevent autolysis (self-dissolving) and have to be activated by special secretions in the stomach and in the duodenum.

The blood carries the products of digestion to the cells where they are either metabolized to yield energy or are involved in synthesis of substances for growth and repair of the organism. Frequent references to glucose level in the blood are called "Blood Sugar Levels." This concentration of glucose in the whole blood remains fairly constant. After 8–12 hours of fasting, the blood-sugar level of a normal adult is usually in the range of 70–90 mg/100 ml blood. Hypoglycemia means the range is below 70 mg/100 ml blood; hyperglycemia denotes any amount above 100 mg/100 ml blood.

Undigested food and secretions are passed from the small intestine to the large intestine by the muscular movements of peristalsis. Numerous bacteria, present in the large intestine, play a part in producing several vitamins, gases and other compounds. As the undigested material moves onward, much of the water is absorbed through the walls of the large intestine. This absorption partially dehydrates wastes (feces) which are eventually eliminated through the rectum and anus at the end of the digestive tract.

The diagram shows that the primary purpose of dietary protein is to furnish amino acids for synthesis of the vast assortment of body proteins. Some amino acids can undergo transamination in order to recombine into other amino acids which can be synthesized by the body (nonessential ones). Unused amino acids are deaminated in the liver and other organs with the amino group changed to urea in the kidney and it with other nitrogenous compounds excreted in the urine. The carbon-hydrogen skeleton can be oxidized to energy or it can be transformed into fat.

The Digestibility of Food

Much confusion exists among the lay public about the meaning of the term, digestibility of food. Is it good for a food to be 100% digestible or is it bad for one to be 50% digestible? Should people eat food of varying digestibility? Is digestibility related to indigestion, poor digestion, or to a "poorly" digested food or meal? Some of the meanings which have been assigned to digestibility include:

1. The percentage of an ingested nutrient or of a diet which was not excreted in the feces is referred to as "coefficient of digestibility" for which mean values are given in Table 5.5, p. 117.
2. The small amount of fecal residue excreted daily or at some other interval of time is compared with the total food intake.
3. The ease and comfort during digestion and during the time following ingestion of a food or meal is often considered in digestibility.

In general, digestibility of food or of a specific nutrient varies with the food, with its processing, or with the individual involved. Factors which have been found to affect digestibility of food include:

1. The higher percentage of cellulose in a food, the lower the digestibility of nutrients, i.e., leaves, stems, and whole seeds have lower percentages of nutrients available for absorption than less fibrous vegetables.
2. The more immature plant structures are lower in cellulose and thus the nutrients are more digestible than those in more mature

structures. In the case of mature seeds the outer bran layers may have been removed in processing as are the peelings of fruits and certain vegetables.

3. In general, cooked plant foods have a higher digestibility of nutrients than raw ones since cooking softens the cellulose allowing the nutrients to be dissolved.

4. Cooking may also change the structure of the nutrient itself such as changes in starch to form dextrins or even some maltose in dry heat treatment.

5. Some animal tissues such as eggs and muscle structures are low in connective tissue and have very high digestibility coefficients. Meats with higher ratio of connective tissue, gristle, and sinews have lower digestibility.

6. Excessive cooking of animal foods, which may be either due to high temperature, to long duration, or to both, definitely reduces the digestibility of the protein in these foods.

7. High fat content especially of fats with high melting points such as tallow derived from suet can reduce digestibility of food containing the fat.

8. The meals themselves affect digestibility. A small volume meal leaves the stomach in 1–3 hours in contrast to a larger volume one which requires 6 or more hours. The composition of the meal and the time interval since the previous food intake affect the time required for digestion. A small meal which consists mostly of carbohydrate-rich foods can be digested in less than 2 hours; e.g., a breakfast consisting of dry toast, fruit juice, and coffee. A higher protein and fat meal consisting of well-buttered toast, sausage, and coffee would take 4 hours or longer to digest and may cause some people to have gastric discomfort or "indigestion."

Activities for Student Learning

1. Read a text on physiology for a better understanding of the digestive process.

2. View a film on digestion such as the "Alimentary Tract."

3. Role-play: Explain digestion to different age groups or to people of different educational levels.

4. Prepare a schematic drawing showing the stages that occur in digestion of a peanut butter sandwich.

5. Some pertinent references are:

   Ingelfinger, F. J. Gastrointestinal absorption, *Nutr. Today*, **2**, 2 (1967).

Mead, J. F. The role of carbohydrates in the diet, *Nutr. Rev.*, **22**, 102 (1964).

Mead, J. F. Metabolic interrelationships of dietary carbohydrate and fat, *Nutr. Rev.*, **22**, 216 (1964).

Mead, J. F. Present knowledge of fat, *Nutr. Rev.*, **24**, 33 (1966).

Mead, J. F. Factors affecting amino acid absorption, *Nutr. Rev.*, **24**, 332 (1966).

Review: Carbohydrate digestion and absorption. *Nutr. Rev.*, **21**, 279 (1963).

6. *Hot Tips:*

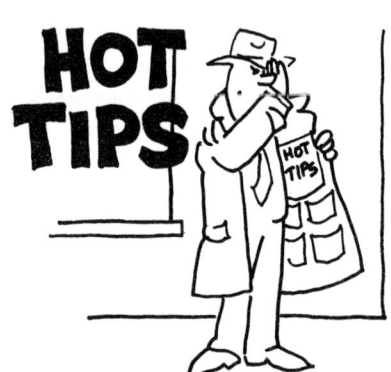

7. *New Words:*

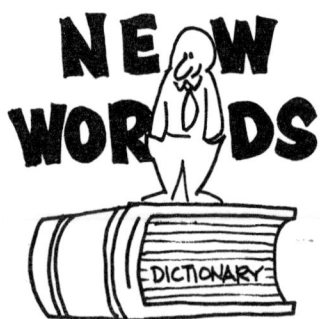

POTENTIAL ENERGY VALUE OF DIETS

Objectives

1. To be able to estimate quickly the approximate calorie content of a food or diet.
2. To be able to decrease or increase the calorie content of certain foods, meals, and diets.

Energy Value of Nutrients

When food is oxidized, energy is released with heat production. The unit of measurement of heat produced by food is termed the large calorie or kilocalorie. This represents the amount of heat required to raise the temperature of 1 kg (2.2 lb) or 1 L (slightly over 1 quart) of water 1°C (from 20° to 21°C). While this unit is correctly designated as a kilocalorie to distinguish it from the smaller unit, a gram calorie (0.001 kcal), many nutritionists refer to it as the Calorie or even just as calorie, assuming that the term is sufficiently standardized for nutrition usage.

A determination of the fuel value of a food may be made in two ways: by computation of energy equivalents of carbohydrates, fats, and proteins, or by direct or indirect calorimetry. Since the body is not 100% efficient in digestion or metabolism, corrections need to be made for values obtained by calorimetry for them to be applicable to people as shown in Table 5.5.

Table 5.5   Energy value of nutrients (kilocalories per gram of nutrient).

	Carbohydrate	Fat	Protein
Heat of combustion:	4.1	9.45	5.65
Less the energy lost by the noncombustion of nitrogen in the body:	0.0	0.0	1.3
Net heat of combustion:	4.1	9.45	4.35
Percentage digested on the average:	98%	95%	92%
Physiological fuel value:	4.0	9.0	4.0
Recommended percentage of calories to be supplied by energy nutrients for the average American diet:	50–60%	30–40%	10–15%

Factors Which Affect the Energy Value of Foods Are

1. The composition or percentage of carbohydrates, fats, and protein present in any given food or diet determines its potential energy value.
2. The percentage of certain noncalorie components in food, either naturally or added in cookery, namely water, cellulose, and air reduce calorie content of the food; e.g., amount of water in a soup, one tablespoon of whipping cream as compared to one of whipped cream, etc.
3. The various procedures in food preparation which include ratios

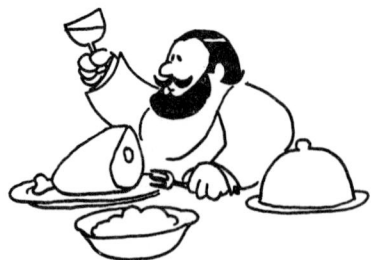

Fig. 5.10 The amount of food eaten depends on a person's concept of the amount of serving.

of fat, sugar and other ingredients used in flour mixtures; e.g., the amount of fat used per cup of flour in making pastry, the amount of fat in meat drippings to make gravy, etc.

4. The addition of seasonings during cooking and the amounts of high calorie items used as fats, bacon, or salt pork, sauces, nuts, cheese, cream, sugar, syrups, and others.

5. The addition of calories at the table such as additional sugar in beverages or on cereal, butter or margarine on breads, vegetables, or potatoes, syrup or jellies on pancakes or breads.

6. The amount of food eaten as a serving which depends on a person's concept of the amount to represent a serving: is it a 12 oz steak or a 4 oz one? a $\frac{1}{8}$ or $\frac{1}{4}$ wedge of pie? 2 or 4 biscuits which are 2 or 3 in. across? cheese with 8 slices in 8 oz package or 12 slices in 8 oz package?

7. The size chosen when food is selected by the unit such as small, medium, or large eggs, apples, oranges, and other unit foods.

8. The nutrient content of substitute or formulated foods such as artificial sweeteners, coffee whiteners, fruit drinks, imitation milk, and the various dessert products.

Foods should be chosen not only to supply calories according to energy needs but they should furnish other nutrients; foods containing mostly calories are said to be sources of *empty* calories. The problem here is really twofold in that empty calorie foods are readily digested leaving a feeling of emptiness and hunger and encouraging excessive calorie consumption. The other aspect of the problem is that either the other nutrients will not be consumed or if they are, the calorie intake will be more excessive. Thus one of the major problems in overeating and overnutrition is making unwise choices in the sources of calories. The supply of empty calorie foods is primarily the product of the food industry since naturally occurring foods are mostly multinutrient in composition.

Modern man is very standardized in his thinking and in his everyday life, except in the food he eats. Eating and cookery even today are haphazard mixtures based on "what I like . . ." in spite of the fact that Fanny Farmer's *Boston Cooking School Cookbook* first published in 1900 had strongly advocated exact measurements in a standard utensil such as a teaspoon, tablespoon, and cup (8 oz); it continued such emphases in all of its 21 editions published prior to her death. Standardization of recipes and serving size greatly influence the adequacy of calorie and nutrient intake. Undoubtedly public eating establishments from the school lunch to the elite club's dining room operate on portion control, standardized recipes, and uniform servings. Food processors, too, are concentrating on "metered calorie" foods. At times industry adds a cheap commodity such as animal fat to a formula and then advertises a "rich" cookie, cake mix, or pastry shell at prices inflated beyond the cost of the added ingredient, and "rich" means high calorie food.

The concept of standardized servings is of vital importance in assuring adequate nutrient and calorie consumption as well as in portion and price control in quantity food production. In order for a given amount of a nutrient to be consumed in adequate amount, the *kind, amount* of food, and the *amount* of additives to a food must be specified.

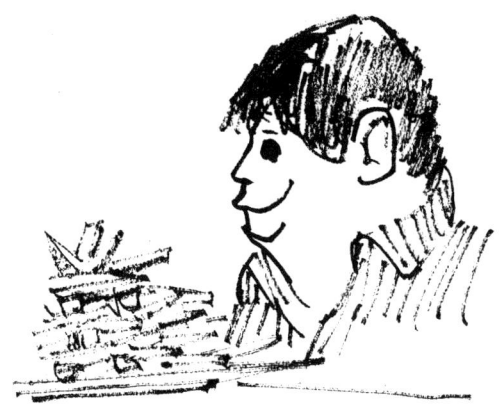

Fig. 5.11 The obese have *NO* concept of standardized servings.

With the multitude of foods and food preparations, to remember average calorie values is very difficult; classification of foods according to calorie value can be easily retained if the principle is understood. The following rule of thumb or guide can be used to estimate the number of calorie in a serving.

Table 5.6   Average calorie value per serving of plain food.

Food Group	Definitely lower than 100 calories (below 75 calories)	Approximately 100 calories (75–125 calories)	Definitely higher than 100 calories (150 calories plus)
Cereal Products	1 slice bread or toast 4 or less 2 in. crackers cereals of large volume for weight (air space)	1 oz of any dry cereal product including ready-to-eat (non-sweetened) ones	1 oz or more of those with added sugar and/or fat
Dairy Products	none, unless serving is less than 1 C milk, 1 oz of cheddar cheese or ½ C cottage cheese	1 C skim milk or buttermilk ½ C cottage cheese 1 T butter (or margarine) 1 oz cheddar cheese	1 C whole milk all products with added sugar and/or fat more than 1 oz of any cheese containing fat
Meats of All Animals	None unless serving is sub-standard, i.e., less than 3 oz of meat; meats devoid of fat as cod and haddock 1 medium or small egg	½ serving (2 oz EP) broiled lean meat 2 oz lean, dried chipped beef 4 oz fish – broiled 1 large egg	Most meats – 4 oz, EP or larger serving
Fruits and Vegetables	½ C cooked or 1 C raw: All leafy All stems (celery) All pods (green beans) All flowers (broccoli) Immature seeds Roots, except potatoes (white or sweet) Most fresh fruit	1 orange, apple, banana, small grapefruit 2–3 peaches ½ C fresh limas 1 small potato (5 oz) 1 oz French Fries ½ C cooked winter squash 5 dates, 3 figs	Nuts high in starch, fat Dried seeds – legumes Sweet potato White potato – large Large servings of sweet fruits All fruits used in pies of various types

Table 5.6 *Continued.*

Food Group	Definitely lower than 100 calories (below 75 calories)	Approximately 100 calories (75–125 calories)	Definitely higher than 100 calories (150 calories plus)

	All berries
	Tomatoes, summer
	  squash, cucumbers,
	  melons, sauerkraut		

Miscellaneous			

	1 T or less of
	  any sweet
		2 T any conc. sweet
		1 T any high fat
		  product, including
		  mayonnaise
		$\frac{2}{3}$ oz potato chips
			Larger amounts of
			  combinations

Food is not good or bad

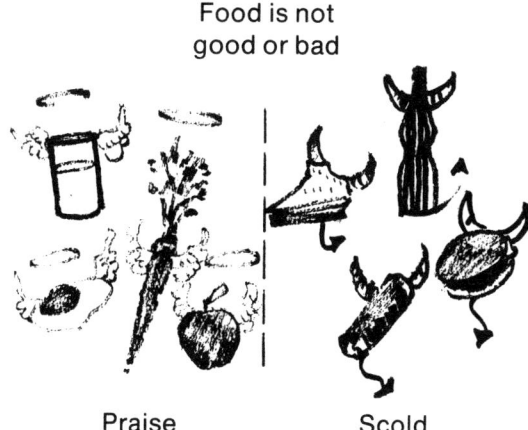

Praise   Scold

Fig. 5.12 Food is neither good nor bad but children may have an image of praise or scold foods.

Activities for Student Learning

1. Study the bar graphs that were prepared when studying the energy nutrients to observe the potential calories of food.
2. Calculate the following problems:
   (a) What is the caloric value of 1 cup (244 g) of milk which contains 3.3% protein, 4.0% fat, 5.0% carbohydrate? What is the caloric value per quart of such milk? What is the influence of serving the same milk after skimming off the cream (fat)?

(b) Calculate the caloric value of 1 (53 g) egg consisting of 11.9% protein, 9.3% fat, 78.8% water. What is the influence of frying this egg in ½ T fat (7 g) which is served with it?

3. Examine foods which show considerable *change in volume* during cooking, such as spinach, cabbage, rice, rolled oats, dried beans and apricots. Weigh 100 calorie size samples of uncooked and cooked food.

4. Examine 100 calorie portion of raw foods which show change in calorie content as a result of cooking, namely bacon, sausage, steak, or other meat in order to determine percentage of calories lost in cooking.

5. List ways in which a cook can add "unseen calories" to a dinner or role-play the teaching of meal planning to adults in order to reduce the number of calories furnished by a meal.

6. Calculate the nutrients in a one-day dietary recall and record as follows:

Calculation of Calories in One-Day Dietary Recall

Food consumer	Amount eaten	Energy value Cal	Nutrient Content—g		
			Protein	Fat	Carbohydrate
Total eaten			—— g	—— g	—— g
Calories/g			× 4	× 9	× 4
Total calories			Cal	Cal	Cal
% of total calories			%	%	%
Recommended distribution of calories			10–15%	30–35%	50–60%
Deviation of intake from recommended					

References and Suggested Readings

Aykroyd, W. R. *Food for Man*. New York: Pergamon, 1969.

Dyke, S. F. *The Carbohydrates*. New York: Interscience, 1960.

Food: An energy exchange system, No. 4 of *The Markets of Change Series*, Kaiser Aluminum and Chemical Corp., Kaiser Center, Oakland, Calif., 1970.

Frazer, A. Doing without the intestine, *Nutr. Today*, **3**: 4, 20 (1968).

Hodges, R. E., and Krehl, W. A. *Effects of Carbohydrates on Lipid Metabolism of Man*. Chicago: Cereal Institute, 1967.

Holt, L. E., *et al*. The concept of protein stores and its implication in the diet, *JAMA*, **181**, 699 (1962).

Ingelfinger, F. J. For want of an enzyme, *Nutr. Today*, **3**: 3, 2 (1968).

Johnson, O. C. Present knowledge of calories (Chapter 1), *Present Knowledge in Nutrition*, 3rd ed. New York: The Nutrition Foundation, 1967.

Markley, K. S. *Fatty Acids*, 2nd ed., Part I. New York: Interscience, 1960.

Mead, J. F. Present knowledge of fat, *Nutr. Rev.*, **24**, 33 (1966).

National Academy of Sciences: Dietary fat and human health, Pub. No. 1147, NRC, Washington, D.C., 1966.

Pigman, W. W., *The Carbohydrates: Chemistry, Biochemistry, Physiology*, New York: Academic Press, 1957.

Programed Instruction for Fat-controlled Diet, 1800 calories, New York: Amer. Heart Assoc., 1969.

Review: Carbohydrate, digestion, and absorption, *Nutr. Rev.*, **21**, 279 (1963).

Sebrell, W. H. It's not age that interferes with nutrition of the elderly, *Nutr. Today*, **1**: 4, 15 (1966).

INVENTORY OF KNOWLEDGE

(Exploration of Concepts in Dietary Supply of Energy)

Part I

The following situations have several solutions proposed. Select the one solution which gives the most relevant and best answer according to recent research:

1. A "fattening food" is best defined as one:
   (a) which contains 100 calories per serving
   (b) which contains at least 250 calories per serving
   (c) any food eaten in excess of body needs
   (d) high in fat content
   (e) a food high in refined carbohydrates

2. Heat, acid, and enzymes hydrolyze starch to:
   (a) glucose, $C_6H_{12}O_6$
   (b) sucrose, $C_{12}H_{22}O_{11}$
   (c) maltose, $C_{12}H_{22}O_{11}$
   (d) cellulose, $(C_6H_{12}O_6)_n$
   (e) amylopectin, $(C_6H_{10}O_5 \cdot H_2O)_n$

3. Primarily carbohydrate comes from plant sources but endogenous carbohydrate may be secured from:
   (a) fats and protein
   (b) vitamins and fats
   (c) minerals and protein
   (d) vitamins and proteins
   (e) cellulose and fats

4. Examples of the most common saturated fatty acids are
   (a) linoleic, linolenic, arachidonic
   (b) linoleic, linolenic, stearic
   (c) stearic, palmitic, linoleic
   (d) stearic, palmitic, myristic
   (e) arachidonic, stearic, palmitic

5. Lipids are essential dietary components because they provide:
   (a) satiety and palatibility of the menu
   (b) padding and insulation for the body
   (c) essential fatty acids
   (d) the most concentrated source of energy and act as a carrier of the fat-soluble vitamins
   (e) all of these

6. Storage of fat in adipose tissue *does not* result from:
   (a) triglycerides
   (b) water intake
   (c) fatty acids
   (d) disaccharides
   (e) amino acids

7. Before protein can be used for energy it must be:
   (a) gelatinized
   (b) fermented
   (c) deaminated
   (d) transaminated
   (e) carbonized

8. The end products of all food oxidized in the body are:
   (a) amino acids, oxygen, and glycerol
   (b) fatty acids, glycerol, and CO_2
   (c) glucose, amino acids, and water
   (d) CO_2, energy, and water
   (e) glucose, calories, and heat

Part II Problem Solving

Apply some of the concepts you have learned in this section and solve the following problems:

9. Mary Jane selected the following foods for breakfast:
   4 oz of orange juice
   1 fried egg
   3 strips of crisp bacon
   1 slice of toast

$\frac{1}{2}$ T of butter on toast

$\frac{1}{2}$ C of skimmed milk

(a) Approximate the total caloric content of breakfast.

(b) If total energy expenditure requires 2000 calories, did her breakfast supply $\frac{1}{3}$–$\frac{1}{4}$ of the day's requirement?

10. Concisely and completely discuss the formation of energy from the three energy nutrients.

6

The Body's Use of Energy

Why the Sudden Concern About Calories and Weight?

During the previous century when "manpower" meant a level of energy expenditure actually expended by a man, calorie intake was measured by hunger and the availability of food. No surplus of calorie consumption occurred for the majority of the people because physical activity was strenuous and food supply variable. Any abundant intake in the summer and fall, which were times of plenty, was inevitably offset by scarcity of food and in many cases subsequent partial starvation during the nonproductive winter months. Any fat deposits were cherished

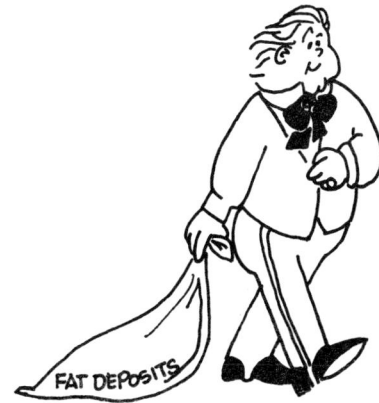

Fig. 6.1 Fatso cherishes his security blanket.

as security against the inevitable disaster which would occur whether it was "natural or man-made." Early man was very insecure in his available food supply. Only a small number of wealthy people were fat, people like Henry VIII or Queen Victoria and a few others whom we see in paintings and read about in the literature.

Especially during the last several decades, more and more people have needed to supply less "manpower" but were required to have more "brainpower" to contribute to their jobs and professions. With this change of emphasis on energy expenditure, no change has occurred in appetite demand.

METABOLISM OF ENERGY IN MAN

Objectives

1. To be able to identify and know the structural parts and processes of the cells found in biological systems.
2. To predict the energy cost of body processes.

The Cell as a Unit for Energy Metabolism

Energy metabolism is the oxidation or combustion which is going on in the animal body during life. The fundamental processes of nutrition take place in the cells. The cell is a structural unit with a boundary or cell membrane consisting of a double wall composed of several alternate layers of protein and lipid substances. The cell membrane determines the transfer of nutrients into the cell. In Fig. 6.2 identification of parts of the cell is shown.

Gross Structures

Cell wall membrane is a flexible covering for the entire cell composed of several layers with different functions.

Cytoplasm contains a variety of structures instrumental in respiration (the mitochondria) and protein synthesis in the ribosomes.

Nucleus is the control center for the cell, the DNA molecules issue chemical instructions to messenger RNA, which transmits the message through the nuclear membrane to the ribosomes.

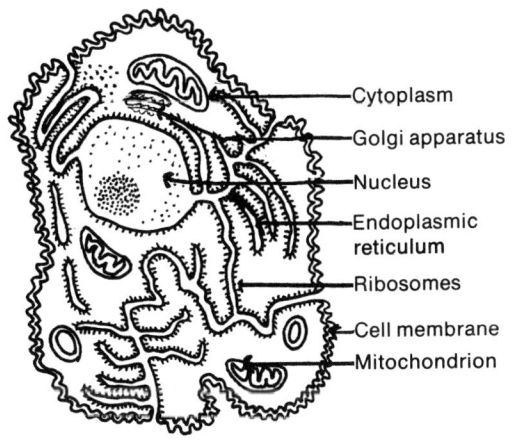

| GROSS STRUCTURES |
| cell wall membranes |
| cytoplasm |
| nucleus |

CYTOPLASMA STRUCTURES
golgi complex
ribosomes
lysosomes
mitochondria
endoplasmic reticulum

CELLULAR FLUIDS
intracellular
intercellular

Fig. 6.2   Diagram of a cell.

Cytoplasmic Structures

Golgi complex is a packet of flat, sacklike membranes, near the nucleus, that stores protein in the form of small granules.

Ribosomes are the site of protein synthesis that is controlled by the messenger RNA which attaches to the surface of the ribosomes.

Endoplasmic reticulum is a network of cavities or channels throughout the cytoplasm that connects with the nuclear membrane and is involved in transfer of molecules and protein synthesis.

Lysosomes are particles enclosing a group of enzymes in a membrane which break down organic molecules into functional units.

Mitochondria represent the areas in which adenosine triphosphate (ATP) the "energy factory" of cellular function is stored.

How do nutrients get inside of cells? Each cell receives nutrients from the surrounding fluids and returns the end product of its metabolic reactions into these same fluids. The molecules are transported through the cell membrane by one of three processes whichever meets the needs:

1. Diffusion is a simple diffusion or movement of molecules from a higher to a lower concentration or gradient with no energy required.
2. Active transport is a movement against a concentration gradient which requires energy to move the molecules.
3. Pinocytosis is a process of the cell membrane enveloping around

something, engulfing by the membrane to take fluids and dissolved substances into the cell; this is probably the process by which virus and bacteria are surrounded.

Which molecules enter a cell? In general, a cell membrane may be either permeable, meaning a substance can pass through it freely; impermeable, meaning a substance cannot pass through it; or semipermeable, meaning some substances can pass, whereas others cannot. Several processes are involved in the transfer of molecules through a cell membrane:

1. Partition coefficient (PC) is the most important determinant; PC is an index of the solubility of a substance in lipids. Compounds that easily dissolve in lipids readily pass through the cell membranes.
2. Molecular size affects transport since smaller molecules enter faster than larger ones provided these have a high partition coefficient.
3. Ionization is the process whereby electrically uncharged molecules enter cells more easily than ions; the electric charge of ions in some manner hinders their passage through the cell membrane.

The activity of cells requires energy and the basic energy system of all cells is a complex system of chemical reactions. Each cell has enzymes in the lysosomes for splitting carbohydrates, fats, and proteins into smaller compounds of glucose, glycerol, fatty acids, and amino acids. The metabolism of these compounds releases tremendous quantities of energy, which is used almost entirely for a single purpose, to convert adenosine diphosphate (ADP) into adenosine triphosphate (ATP). The ATP molecule then supplies the needed energy to the different chemical reactions required in the life of the cell.

Reactions for Release of Energy

The general reaction to represent the release of energy can be presented as follows where the first half is the anaerobic reaction with limited energy release (2 ATP) and the second half involving respiration with the production of 36 ATP:

$$C_6H_{12}O_6 \longrightarrow 2 \text{ pyruvate and 2 ATP} \longrightarrow \text{acetyl coenzyme A}$$
glucose

$$\text{acetyl coenzyme A} + 6O_2 \longrightarrow 36 ATP + 6H_2O + 6CO_2$$

Specifically two stages occur in this generalization, the first is an anaerobic respiration or glycolysis reaction in which the initiation of energy metabolism yields 2 ATP per mole of glucose. The second stage is described as aerobic respiration or Krebs cycle which is also called the citric cycle or tricarboxylic acid cycle (TCA cycle):

$$C_6 \rightarrow C_3 + C_3 \rightarrow \text{pyruvic acid} \rightarrow \underset{\text{coenzyme A}}{\text{acetyl}} \rightarrow \underset{\text{cycle}}{\text{Krebs}} \rightarrow 36 \text{ moles } ATP + H_2O + CO_2$$

The adenosine triphosphate molecule (ATP) is a nucleotide composed of the nitrogenous base, adenine, the pentose sugar, ribose, and three molecules of phosphoric acid. When adenosine triphosphate releases its energy, a phosphoric acid radical is split away and adenosine diphosphate (ADP) is formed. ADP plus 1 phosphoric acid can then be recombined by the anaerobic and aerobic processes to form a new adenosine triphosphate, the entire process continuing over and over again.

ATP supplies energy used to promote three major categories of cellular functions (1) membrane transport, (2) synthesis of chemical compounds throughout the cell, and (3) performance of mechanical work. ATP is always available to release its energy rapidly and almost explosively wherever it is needed in the cell. The cell uses energy from 3 sources which is shown in Table 6.1.

Table 6.1 Pathways of energy metabolism.

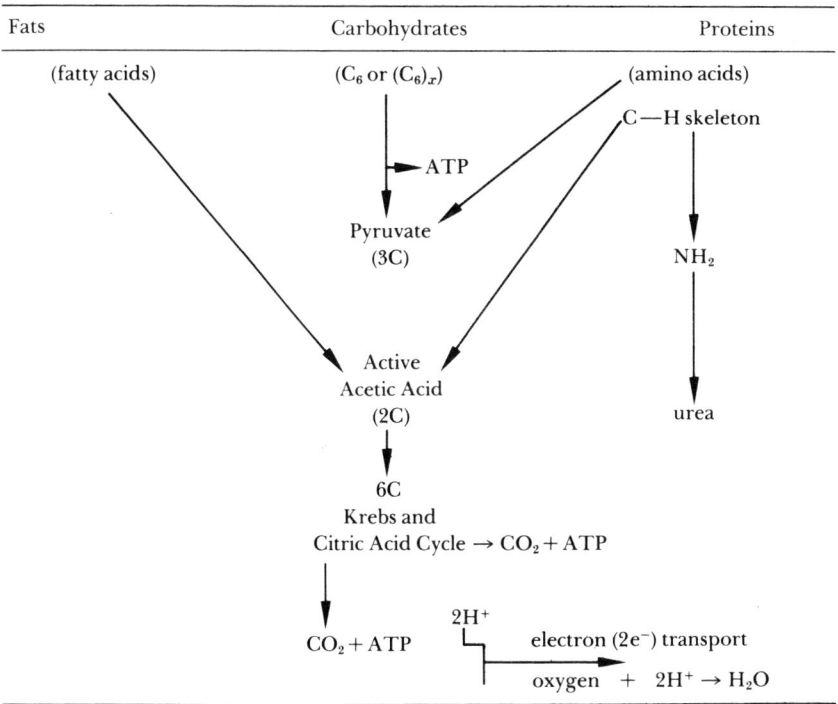

Fats	Carbohydrates	Proteins
(fatty acids)	$(C_6 \text{ or } (C_6)_x)$	(amino acids)

Pyruvate (3C)

Active Acetic Acid (2C)

6C
Krebs and
Citric Acid Cycle $\rightarrow CO_2 + ATP$

$CO_2 + ATP$

C—H skeleton

NH_2

urea

$2H^+$
electron (2e⁻) transport
oxygen + $2H^+ \rightarrow H_2O$

Activities for Student Learning

1. Supplement your understanding of the production of energy by further reading.
2. Explain the physiological or chemical processes which are implied in Fig. 6.3.
3. Sketch a model of a cell, identifying the role of the component parts in nutrition.

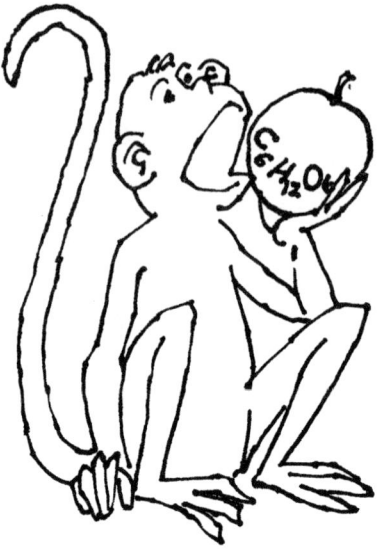

Fig. 6.3 ... "any kind of animal."

FACETS OF ENERGY EXPENDITURE

Objectives

1. To identify energy as a measurable quantity in human life and to estimate accurately the basal energy needed by living tissue during growth and activity.
2. To be able to compute the calorie balance for any given individual recognizing positive calorie balance during growth, zero calorie balance during adulthood, and negative calorie balance on reducing regimen.

Body Composition

A summary of the factors involved in body composition is essential to understanding the body's need for energy. The different tissues have different energy levels with muscle mass constituting the major portion of energy expenditure of the body even under resting conditions.

The body exhibits a remarkable "compositional homeostasis." This constancy in an individual person is established by his genetic code, his hormone balance, and his uniform pattern of living, but can be altered by his activity patterns, dietary regimen, age, disease, medical treatment, and pregnancy. The individual is also influenced by his environmental temperature. Improved methodology to determine accurately body composition during infancy, childhood, adolescence, adulthood, and old age is very important to defining optimal nutritional needs for each of these phases of life.

Substantial advances have been made in the past two decades in technics for studying body composition in a variety of experimental, clinical, and epidemiological contexts. Total body water as percentage of body weight is highest during fetal life and decreases with advancing age. Water retention is a major factor in daily fluctuation of body weight. Differences in body composition between the male and female are evident early in life but become most pronounced at sexual maturity. The male generally contains a greater percentage of body weight

Self-appraisal

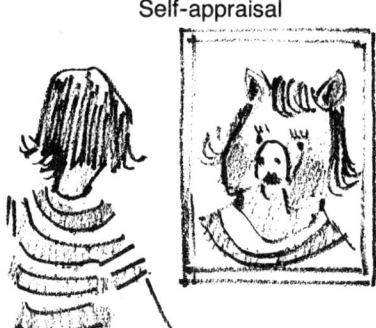

Fig. 6.4 Self-appraisal can be very misleading, especially when done by adolescent girls themselves.

as fat-free tissue, whereas the female is more prone to adiposity. Diet and exercise patterns influence body composition at any age.

Research methods by J. Brozek are used to identify body composition; such methods may be summarized under the following titles:

Densitometric methods are used to estimate the variable quantity of body fat. From these measurements emerged the concept of lean body mass which is determined by difference of the whole body mass minus non-essential or excess lipids. Lean body mass differs from the fat-free body in that essential structural lipids are included. Since the density of fat is less than that of other body components, as the percentage of body fat increases, the total body density decreases. Expense, time, difficulties, and restrictions encountered in measuring body density by hydrometry have led to the development of measuring body composition by other methods including gasometric ones using helium-air displacement procedures.

Dilution methodology is based on the concept that certain substances distribute themselves evenly within a specific body water compartment and that the dilution of a known amount of substance introduced into an unknown volume permits calculation for that unknown volume. Antipyrine is a substance which disperses evenly throughout the total body water and can be used for determining the total body water; injected thiocynate and inulin permit measurement of extracellular water. The difference in amounts between the total body water and extracellular water indicates the amount of intracellular water.

Roentgenographic methods using low intensity irradiation differentiate the width of the subcutaneous fat layer from muscle and skin. This method produces results comparable to skin fold measurements.

Radioactive elements such as Potassium[40] to identify the fat-free body mass promises to be a realistic approach to the study of body composition since potassium is concentrated in body cells other than those of adipose tissue.

Obviously none of these methods are practical for use in a doctor's office or by an individual to assess his own body composition. A pressing need exists for a practical, reasonably precise and reproducible method to estimate body composition. Body weight, being a sum of low-fat body tissue and total body fat, does not reflect body composition. Skin fold thicknesses are more reliable indices of total body fat. The triceps skin fold is the "best simple predictor of body density (and hence percentage total body fat)" in obese adolescent girls and is a "practical and accurate estimate of adiposity" in the adolescent body. Self-appraisal without data can result in major misconceptions.

The concepts of body composition and analysis of body size are more fully presented in Section 3.

Basal Metabolism as a Portion of Daily Energy Expenditure

Basal metabolism is defined as the least amount of energy required for the body to live while awake. This may be compared to paying rent on a business building, regardless of whether the sales are good or bad, the rent expense must be paid; or it is like the motor running when the car is not going anywhere, but it has to be ready to move. Basal metabolism is expressed in kilocalories per kilogram body weight or per square meter of surface area. In spite of the variation in fat content, body weight and surface area correlate closely with heat production.

Heat is lost from the body under normal conditions; only when illness interferes with heat loss, does the body retain excess heat in the condition described as fever. Heat production must equal heat losses from the body to maintain a constant normal body temperature characteristic of the human being. Therefore, heat losses can be measured in methods of direct calorimetry to indicate energy transformations; naturally respiratory exchange has to be included. Measurement of direct calorimetry is very complicated requiring much costly equipment and highly trained researchers. By the early 1920s equipment had been designed to measure the respiratory exchange without considering heat production. Since the amount of oxygen uptake and carbon dioxide production are only indirectly related to heat production, respiration measurements are referred to as indirect calorimetry. Many nutrition textbooks have a good discussion of the equipment, procedure, and various aspects of basal metabolism.

Conditions under which a person is said to be expending energy at a *basal metabolic rate* (BMR) have been described as:

lying down in the most comfortable environment;
awake, since relaxed sleep is approximately 10% lower;
postabsorptive state achieved by 12–14 hours after the last food intake
    such as can occur prior to breakfast in the morning;
relaxed muscles, limited tension and without mental anxiety.

The attempt is to measure the lowest level of energy expenditure of a person while awake in order to assess the energy cost of the body "doing nothing" but living; this may be compared to a motor which "idles" whenever it is not in gear to do work.

Obviously, many factors cause variations in this basal energy metabolic rate. From 1900 to about the 1930s frequent research treatises were published. During the last few decades little research has been reported on gross metabolic activity of the human body but studies have concentrated on cellular biochemistry. The general factors to affect the basal energy metabolic rate are as valid in the 1970s as when they were proposed prior to the 1920s.

Basal metabolic rate is dependent on body size as indicated by weight, or more accurately defined as surface area which is more indicative of volume than weight alone. Since body temperature is a relatively constant value within one or two degrees of the mean of 98°F, heat production has to be proportional to the rate of heat losses during normal life. The tall, slender body looses heat faster and would have a higher BMR than the short stocky person who may weigh the same as the tall one.

Age is a factor of major significance in its implications in human nutrition. The newborn's basal metabolism rises rapidly in proportion to the rate of growth (three times the initial body size) and to the development of muscles and their control during one year's life-span. The child reaches his life's apex of basal heat production at about two years of age. Then gradually the rate decreases until the period of early adolescence when another rise occurs. After the puberty rise, the BMR gradually decreases throughout the adult period, about 10–15% from early adulthood to age 75 years. The changes in BMR during the life-span account for the fact that children are warm and object to wraps when adults feel cool; this accounts for a definition told in nursery school, "a sweater is a wrap a child wears when the teacher feels cold." Figure 6.5 shows the changes in BMR with age.

By the beginning of adolescence, sex differences in basal heat production occur; first the girls show the prepuberty rise about two years younger than boys. When the boys reach the puberty stage of

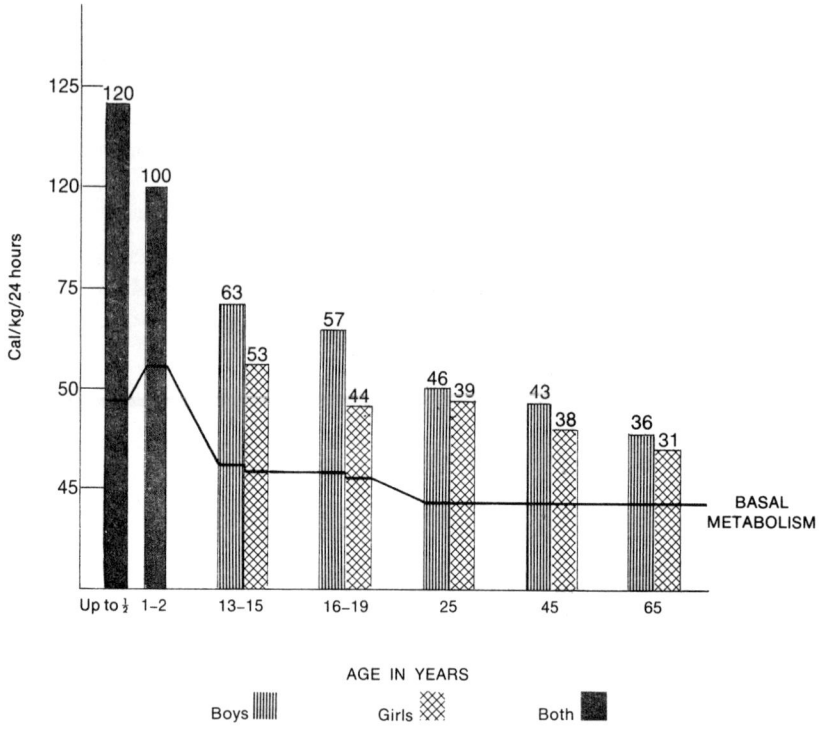

Fig. 6.5 A comparison of estimated energy expenditure and basal metabolism. The data show the high calorie expenditure of infants and adolescents in contrast to that of adults and the proportion of expenditure required for basal metabolism in contrast to that required for activity.

development, their basal energy expenditure exceeds that of the girls and continues to be higher per unit of body weight or surface area throughout the life-span. This difference is attributed to the greater muscularity of men and their greater lean body mass with their lower percentage of adipose tissue than in the bodies of women. This difference in body composition is also noted to be characteristic of the two sexes of other animals, such as cattle, chickens, and hogs when their carcasses are evaluated for yield of edible meat.

Other factors often discussed include the influence of wide variations in climate, especially temperatures, racial, and cultural influences including contrasts in dietary intake dominant in carbohydrates or in protein by various people of the world.

Currently, basal metabolic rates are seldom determined in medical diagnosis; the medical laboratory has developed the measurement of protein bound iodine (PBI) as indicative of thyroxin activity, a hormone of thyroid gland. Relationship of thyroxin function and basal heat production has long been recognized but no numerical ratio has been established. Other hormones are also involved in BMR; adrenalin under stress increases blood sugar supplies and raises heat production; excessive insulin may lower blood sugar, producing hypoglycemia.

Basal metabolism, expressed as kilocalories per unit of body size, shows a remarkable uniformity between individual persons of similar size and age ranges. For practical use adults can conveniently predict their own basal metabolism from data of early research by Harris and Benedict from Carnegie Nutrition Laboratory, who determined the basal heat production to be equal to one calorie for each kilogram of "normal" body weight for each hour. This relationship is usually expressed as:

$$BMR = 1 \text{ Cal/kg/hr.}$$

Persons who deviate from their recommended weight for height, frame size, and sex, should use the recommended weight, rather than their own, in estimating their basal metabolism.

Total Energy Expenditures

The total energy expenditure of the body depends on its size and composition, and on the level and duration of activity. The energy cost of work depends on the number of muscles involved, the duration of the activity, the speed or rate of movement, and the total strength exerted. Running, for example, may require a higher or lower expenditure of calories per hour than walking, depending on the speed required for the best muscle coordination for that individual. Table 6.4 (p. 143) illustrates the relationship between the calorie content of various amounts of foods and the time required to spend these calories in different activities.

Determining the exact number of calories expended daily by the average individual is difficult and time-consuming. In order to calculate quickly the energy for different individuals, estimation pertaining to categories of sedentary, moderate, active or severe activity can be employed as shown in Table 6.2. Research surveys show that the activity level differs for those who are obese or slender as shown in Fig. 6.6.

Table 6.3 shows certain characteristics that can be related to the predicted energy expenditure of people in the life-cycle. For example, calorie needs per kilogram of body weight per day for the rapidly

Table 6.2 Simplified estimate of energy expenditure.

Daily level of exertion	Description of daily activity	Calorie cost per day		
		per kg	Woman 58 kg	Man 70 kg
Sleep	lying down comfortably, relaxed muscles, postabsorptive state	22	1276	1540
			10% less than BMR	
Awake (BMR)	lying down comfortably, relaxed muscles, postabsorptive state	24	1400	1700
Very light (sitting – sedentary)	muscles hold body with support, limited movement, mostly sitting and some walking, low muscle tone	30	1690	2040
			BMR + 20% activity	
Light (standing)	muscles hold body erect, movement in one plane, activity mostly sitting or standing, casual walking with little stress	34	2160	2380
			BMR + 40% activity	
Moderate (more active)	more large muscles used in multi-movements, some stressful activity (1–2 hr), activity to stress muscles for 3–5 hr	38	2240	2560
			BMR + 60% activity	
Activity (longer periods of activity)	much total body muscle use, more vertical and stressful, exertion for 4–6 hr, maximum for very active woman	43	2520	3000
			BMR + 80% activity	
Very active	Total body use for 12 hr, stressful exertion for 8 hr, well-muscled build required	Above 48	Doubtful	Above 3500

Activity?

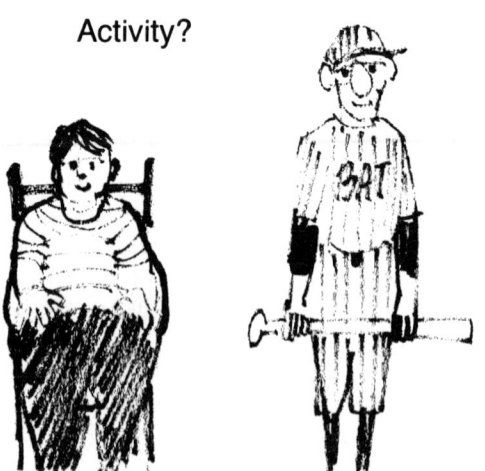

Fig. 6.6 The obese adolescent is less active than the nonobese.

Table 6.3   Predicted energy expenditures of people in the life-cycle based on 1968 revised NRC's RDA.

Age range years	Characteristics related to energy expenditures	Wt. range kg	Cal/kg/day
Infant 0–1	most rapid rate of growth development of muscle strength, high rate of heat production, great amount of total body movement for each activity appetite demands 3–4-hour interval eating schedule	4–9	120–100
1–6	reduced rate of growth, continued increase in muscle strength, heat production related to quieter activity movement restricted to fewer muscles involved in activity, reduced appetite increases time between meals and less food eaten per unit of size	12–19	90–87
6–10	continued slower growth rate, increased muscle strength, activities involve the total body such as wrestling, football, etc. increased appetite associated with activity	23–28	87–78
10–14	accelerated growth differs in sexes, growth seems disproportionate, i.e., large feet and hands, long legs or arms in proportion to size of body increased pads of subcutaneous fat, i.e., breasts, hips, stomach, activity variable and appetite erratic, tremendous, and none	35–43 boys 35–44 girls	71–63 boys 64–52 girls
14–18	difference in sex; girls attain mature size but boys continue to grow activity variable and erratic, related to sex	59 boys 52–54 girls	51 boys 42–43 girls
18–22	stabilized weight and body composition (adult type), high muscle tone and strength highest ratio of protein in tissue, good appetite; food consumption dependent on familial pattern, occupation, and social eating	67 men 58 women	42 men 35 women
22–55 prime adult	continued stable weight depends on continued activity, good appetite; eating depends on occupation and social customs	70 men 58 women	40–38 men 35–32 women
55–75+	weight may be constant but increased proportions of fat in tissues replaces protein, reduced muscle tone and strength reduced heat production, moderate appetite and eating due to customary practice	70 men 58 women	34 men 29 women

developing infant are approximately four times higher than those for the adult.

Activities for Student Learning

1. What is metabolism? What happens to the rate of metabolism during physical activity? How does this affect body temperature? How is shivering related to metabolism?
2. Where and what is the hypothalamus? What effect does it have on the temperature of the body? What would happen to the body if the hypothalamus were injured?
3. Study pictures of persons engaged in different physical activities. How many muscles are involved? Are the muscles being used to maximum strength?

ENERGY BALANCE AND WEIGHT CONTROL

Objectives

1. To identify factors which may affect the food intake of an individual as related to energy balance and adiposity.
2. To implement procedures to prevent the accumulation of undesirable adipose tissue.
3. To compare sources of calories in an individual's choice of food, the quantity eaten, and seasonings added.

The Meanings of Energy Balance

Energy balance may be defined as zero, positive, or negative balance. *Zero balance* indicates that "input equals output," the energy value of food eaten is equivalent to energy expenditure, and the weight of the individual remains stationary. *Positive energy* balance means that "input exceeds output," more calories are consumed than expended, the extra calories are stored as glycogen in the liver, then as fat in adipose cells; in general one pound of adipose tissue may be formed when 3500 extra calories are consumed beyond

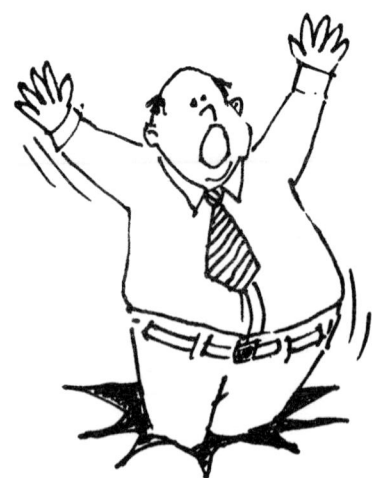

Fig. 6.7 Obesity has far-reaching detrimental effects on health.

the energy needs. However, positive energy balance is necessary for periods of growth, during childhood, adolescence, and during pregnancy and lactation, in addition to recovery from disease or in muscle development during training for physical performance.

Negative balance means that the "input is less than the output," a type of negative spending when more energy is used than was supplied by the food, body tissues have to supply the deficit. A point in weight loss can occur when cells can no longer supply the energy required for life and "the body starves to death." No other nutrients can supply the energy needed except carbohydrates, fats, and proteins; these come either from food or from tissues of the body itself. In a negative calorie balance, either the input is too limited or the output is excessive. This leads to deterioration of body tissue; the liver stores of glycogen become marginal, fat mobilization exceeds fat synthesis, and the protein content of tissues is decreased. Protein molecules will be deaminated, the carbon-hydrogen skeleton will be used for energy and the nitrogen is excreted as urea. Thus urinary nitrogen is indicative of protein breakdown due to insufficient intake of energy or excessive intake of protein. When this occurs, physiological disturbances are apt to occur such as retarded growth and depressed synthesis of enzymes and hormones.

Regulation of Food Intake

Any intake of energy nutrients above that needed to meet the energy requirements results in the storage, first of glycogen, and then of body depot fat. This is a useful survival factor in wild animals since they can store fat during a season of plentiful food as a reserve against the relative starvation of the winter season. During past decades, "fat wives" were prized possessions as they would be "more likely to live during a time of famine."

Hunger and appetite sensations prompt a man or animal to consume food. Hunger may be considered physiological in that multiple autonomic responses to the changes in blood sugar stimulate centers in the hypothalamus. When blood glucose concentrations are lowered, this will cause stomach contractions which are associated with extreme hunger. Research results showed that caged dogs ate more than noncaged, and that a "lean" person has "stomach clock regulators," whereas a fat person has increased sensory perception to odors and sights of food which causes increased hunger sensations.

Appetite in man is a complicated response based on psychological and physiological factors. The psychological factors are extremely complex determinants of what we accept as food and whether to eat it at any prescribed time. Interestingly, the response to a stimulus may be the opposite in different persons, one may eat twice as much of an acceptable food and the other may have an aversion to eating any of the food under those circumstances. Furthermore, at one time a person may eat food and under a different stimulus, he may refuse.

The kind of food served, the standards of cooking, the temperature of the food and of the environment, and the setting for eating, whether solitary, happy, domestic, or social all affect a person's desire to eat. Habit also plays a part in the regulation of food intake. People become accustomed to a "feeling of fullness." The time factor is obvious with the idea of three meals per day served "on time;" many eat by the clock. Familial values become apparent in any analysis of food patterns; culture, customs, religion, and environment—rural versus urban, pleasant versus unpleasant—affect the acceptance of food and the amount consumed. Also, feelings of rejection are coupled with sensations of hunger and may affect food intake in opposite extremes, gluttony or anorexia.

The "glucostatic" theory postulates that, depending on the kind of psychological conditioning listed above, satiety results from a complex of interrelation between glucose level, its rate of utilization, and the rate of storage. Specific and minute lesions made experimentally in the hypothalamus of rats lead to tremendous overeating (hyperphagia) and those in other nearby points of the hypothalamus lead to refusing to eat (hypophagia).

Research with laboratory rats has shown that mature rats will ordinarily regulate their food intake so that their body weight remains about constant. The day-to-day intake of food by the rats may vary considerably, but over a period of one or more weeks little variation occurs. Unfortunately, all humans do not always demonstrate this characteristic; however, the precision with which food intake is regulated is obvious in many people. In the course of 25 years of varied activity, a man can eat 12 tons of food and yet have a variation of only 2–3 pounds weight. In people, food consumption is regulated by the appetite of the individual, food availability, and by socioeconomic factors. Of course, in some parts of the world, the limit on food intake is rigidly set and/or limited by the amount of food available, whether it can be grown, purchased, or foraged by the family.

Various attempts have been made to correlate the potential energy value of a given amount of food and the metabolic cost of standardized exercises and activities. Such comparisons have many assumptions and pitfalls for interpretation. Konishi (1965) presented data which are given in Table 6.4, calculated on the basis of 70 kg weight of young men.

Data in Table 6.4 for dairy products illustrate that individual foods differ and that the amount of the food eaten determines its calorie content. In general, a man is thought to work an eight hour schedule at a rate of 5 Cal/min/70 kg man or 2400 Cal/8 hr schedule/70 kg man. Whether women can expend energy at this rate is doubtful since the percentage of adipose tissue reduces the metabolic rate per kilogram body weight. The data could not be simply recalculated to apply to the average 58 kg woman. Since a man is heavier, the cost of energy for an identical activity would differ.

According to Sparge (1966), obese adolescents are more common in middle income families than in

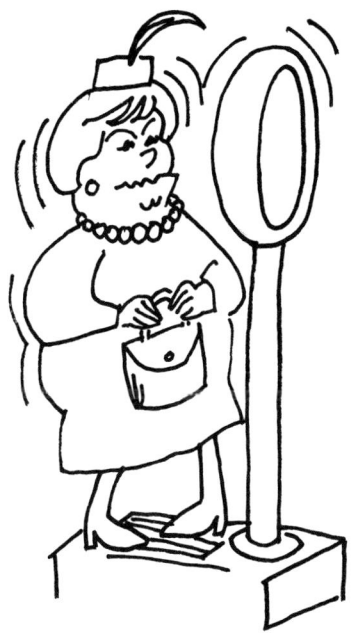

Fig. 6.8 "Oh-h----how did this happen? The scale must be broken."

Table 6.4 Energy equivalents of food calories.

| Food — amount | Calories | Activity in minutes | | | | |
		(1) Reclining	(2) Walking	(3) Bicycling	(4) Swimming	(5) Running
Milk, 1 C	166	128	32	20	15	9
Skim milk, 1 C	81	62	16	10	7	4
Milk shake, 12 oz	421	324	81	51	38	22
Ice milk, $\frac{1}{6}$ qt	144	111	28	18	13	7
Sherbet, $\frac{1}{6}$ qt	177	136	34	22	16	9
Ice cream, $\frac{1}{6}$ qt	193	148	37	24	17	10
Cottage cheese, 1 T	27	21	5	3	2	1
Cheddar cheese, 1 oz	111	85	21	14	10	6

(1) Reclining at 1.3 Cal/min/70 kg man or only slightly above BMR
(2) Walking at 3.5 mph or 5.2 Cal/min/70 kg man
(3) Bicycling at 8.2 Cal/min/70 kg man
(4) Swimming at 11.2 Cal/min/70 kg man
(5) Running at 19.4 Cal/min/70 kg man

the high or low income families. Stunkard (1962) and her co-workers found a level of obesity seven times higher than average among women reared in the lower socioeconomic strata. A lesser percentage was found in men.

Many factors modify the normal energy balance. Obesity is not a single disease entity but is a symptom of an underlying energy imbalance that may have many causes. The "disease" is best tackled by looking for the causes which may be:

I. Physiological — Controversy exists as to the efficiency of food utilization and the enzymatic differences which cause individual variations. Mobilization of fat may be relatively slow, therefore physical activity rapidly depletes the carbohydrate stores causing hunger without draining upon the fat reserves. Genetic factors may be the principal determinants for some obese individuals. Disorders have been identified as well as relationships that exist between the hypothalamus and other cerebral centers; ultimately these complexities of the central regulatory mechanisms will probably be unraveled to improve the understanding of the pathogenesis of some forms of obesity.

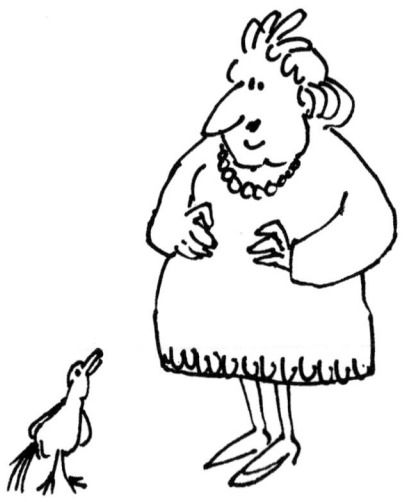
Fig. 6.9   "I eat like a bird."

The phrase "fat and forty" has a basis for truth when considering the steadily reduced BMR for this aged individual. This can be said to be an endocrine disorder of aging, but the glands of internal secretion are only partly responsible for aging and for the distribution of body fat. Women deposit excess fat in the areas of the hips, thighs, buttocks, breasts, and back of the neck called a "dowagers hump." In men, the accumulation of fat occurs in the neck and the abdominal region; this is often termed a "bay window." People, as well as other animals, fatten with increased age up to about age 65 years. Dr. Jean Mayer believes that the role of genetic factors in the obesities should be recognized and used in anticipating obesity rather than resignation to an obvious fate. Children of obese parents are more likely to become obese; therefore, preventative measures such as proper food, exercise habits, and recognition of factors involved should be taught early.

II. Sociological causes (socioeconomic level and family environment) –
Obesity in man to an extraordinary degree is under the control of social
factors such as customs developed in the days of physical exertion. Within the family environment, members may be faced with the development
of the habit to overeat which encourages the children of obese parents to
overeat. Feelings of warmth, solidarity, and love become associated with
certain foods. Certainly, the presence of such modern labor-saving
devices as the washing machine, vacuum cleaners, single story homes,
dishwashers, wash and wear clothing, etc. reduce the amount of energy
expended. In addition, an abundance of food is available at any time of
the day. The tendency "don't walk anywhere, when you can ride" is
impressed on children, and advertising influences the choices, likes and
dislikes of everyone. Other familial influences or overtones may be:
(a) Is food used for rewards or companionship? (b) Are all servings
"overly" generous? (c) What is considered "good" food in the family
functions? Is it carrot sticks or a serving of chocolate cake? (d) Is it more
thrifty to eat all the leftovers, "the clean plate club," or to discard them?
and (e) Is television viewing the favorite pastime or is it participation
in work and play? Thus family food patterns resulting from past history,
religious or ethnic customs are "set" in children for their lifetime.

III. Psychological – An obese child usually remains obese all of his
life; his emotional life centers around eating, avoiding physical activity,
and many social contacts. In the North American society, the obese individual is often identified as undesirable, unhealthy, and definitely
not the lean stereotype image of health, beauty, and desirability that the
public accepts. Often, boredom culminates in nibbling and eating even
when the person is not really hungry. Hyperphagia or overeating may
be sporadic and in response to frustration. Such a condition may be
recognized as the "night-eating syndrome," but is probably the most
clear-cut example of the utilization of food as a substitute for love or
self-respect. Obesity may be acquired by an adolescent girl as a guarantee
against dating. The fat person essentially retires from sexual competition
and this may be an important subconscious motivation in overeating.

Hazards of energy imbalance or complications due to obesity are
numerous. There is a relationship between health and weight; the risk
to health can increase with added pounds. Experts report that it is point-
less to lose or gain weight unless the individual intends to maintain a
desirable weight.

With excess weight, a greater burden is placed on the heart and the
circulatory system, especially when muscular exertion is increased. Some
problems that may affect the overweight person include: arterial hyper-

tension and high blood pressure, increased sweating since fat below the skin prevents efficient escape of heat, increased labor of breathing, difficulty in ambulation especially with diseases such as arthritis or recovery from fractures, and disfigurement (poor stomach alignment, crowded digestive area, etc.). Other resulting problems include certain diseases such as gall bladder disease, gout, diabetes mellitus, hypertension, and possibly coronary atherosclerosis, metabolic disorders of the pancreas and liver, psychic trauma, increased surgical risks and more prone to accidents, diminished longevity, and increased mortality.

What is the secret to the management of obesity? "One recipe for long life is never exceed the feed limit." The prevention of obesity is really the first and only good solution to the problem. Preventive measures must be built to attack the underlying causes for the development of obesity, whether they be cultural, psychological, sociological, metabolic, economic, genetic, or environmental. The greatest hope lies with oncoming generations in which a key role in prevention of obesity should be played by physicians, obstetricians, nutritionists, public school teachers, social scientists, public health workers, and *Mothers*.

The second solution is to maintain the *status quo*, not to allow weight to fluctuate. Basically, choosing the proper foods and balancing this calorie intake with activity pays dividends in a healthful long life.

The third solution is to undertake some form of weight reduction which is most likely to succeed during the early stages of obesity. Obesity acquired as an adult is easier to reduce than that of an adult who was obese as a child. Special reducing technics which may be employed include possessing the desire to reduce, developing the motivation by family support and understanding, possessing a reasonable degree of emotional stability, and joining organizations that support and encourage people to lose weight. Regular physical activity should be increased rather than sporadic bursts of activity. The best type of exercise is to push away from the table at the right time. Eating habits should be regulated and modified to include eating slowly, selecting smaller *size* servings, preparing foods in such ways as to reduce the caloric content, and avoiding fad diets and diet pills.

A peculiar malady that affects many Americans is "diet-itis." Everyone is diet conscious, "on a diet," "going on one," or "just finished a diet." Many overweight Americans are malnourished due to poor food choices; following of fad diets can only aggravate the problem. The only solution is planning and eating good meals that keep the nutrient intake "up" and the calories "down." Individuals need to control weight, not by dieting, but by not overeating, plus, a daily exercise regimen built into the normal routine of living.

Just as fads in fashions come and go, fad diets come and go. Through the years many fads have been associated with weight reducing. Once

Table 6.5   Ten calorie diet.

Monday:
  Breakfast — Weak Tea
  Lunch   — 1 Bouillon Cube in ½C Diluted Water
  Dinner   — 1 Pigeon Thigh & 3 oz Prune Juice

Tuesday:
  Breakfast — Scraped Crumbs from Burnt Toast
  Lunch   — Doughnut Hole (w/o sugar) & 1 Glass Dehydrated Water
  Dinner   — Canary Eyebrows Stewed (Fat Removed)

Wednesday:
  Breakfast — Boiled Out Stains of Tablecloth
  Lunch   — One-Half Dozen Poppy Seeds
  Dinner   — Bee's Knees & Mosquito Knuckles Sauted with Vinegar

Thursday:
  Breakfast — Shredded Egg-Shell Skins
  Lunch   — Belly Button from A Naval Orange
  Dinner   — Three Eyes from Irish Potato (Diced)

Friday:
  Breakfast — Four Chopped Banana Seeds
  Lunch   — Broiled Butterfly Liver
  Dinner   — Fillet of Soft Shell Crab Claw

Saturday:
  Breakfast — Two Lobster Antennae
  Lunch   — One Guppy Fin
  Dinner   — Jelly Fish Vertebrae *à la* Bookbinder

Sunday:
  Breakfast — Pickled Humming Bird Tongue
  Lunch   — Prime Ribs of Tadpole
  Dinner   — Tossed Paprika & Clover Leaf (one salad only)

Directions: 1. All meals to be eaten under microscope to avoid extra portions.
               2. Second Week: Reversed
               3. Third Week: Funeral (Choice of Directors)

Source Unknown

there was Fletcherizing or chewing each mouthful of food 32 times; other dietary regimens to avoid include the:

Hollywood Eighteen Day Diet	Banana Diet
Egg Diet	Three-day Diet
All-meat Diet	Calories Don't Count
Drinking Man's Diet	Zen No Fruit Diet (no fruit, no
Mayo Reducing Diet	meat, no milk)
Grapefruit Diet	Grape Juice Diet
Starvation Diet or Complete	The Steak Diet
Fasting	The Pennington Diet
The "fat" Diet	Ten Calorie Diet (Table 6.5)

The very multiplicity of fad diets is a testimony to their ineffectiveness. Most of them tend to be based on the idea, that with the Proper diet, "calories don't count" — an idea which is nutritionally absurd but appeals to those who would like to "eat their cake and reduce, too!"

The free use of empty calories is the main cause of hyperphagia. The average American eats 500 calories per day from sugar, 600 calories per day from visible fats, and 125 calories per day from alcoholic beverages. These calories total over 1200 calories per day; about 40% of the total daily intake. Consumptions of one hundred excess calories per day will result in about ten pounds of extra weight within one year. For every pound that one is overweight, life expectancy is decreased approximately forty days.

Nutritionally adequate diets are the only answer to the selection of the "best diet." The Food and Nutrition Board, National Academy of Sciences of the National Research Council has suggested that the normal adult requires approximately 500 calories from carbohydrate daily, and one gram of protein per kilogram of body weight per day for adults of all ages. No specific recommendation has been made for fat. The conclusion is that a varied diet is the best one: choose the proper amounts from the four food groups.

Activities for Student Learning

1. Study selected references concerning weight control and analyze methods used to motivate people to lose weight in one to one teaching and in group therapy. Identify technics which aid people to reeducate their food and eating habits.
2. Assume that you are a nutritionist in public health, a hospital or clinical dietitian, a teacher of health, or a nurse. How would you advise someone or a group who needs to control body weight?

Design a plan for such an instruction unit.

3. Study the principles involved in the group therapy applied in national organizations for weight control such as "TOPS" and "Weight-Watchers." Calculate the protein/calorie ratio used in their diet recommendations.

4. Design the general structure and counseling service which would be most effective with weight loss in obese individuals who are:
   (a) children to early adolescents,
   (b) teenagers,
   (c) young homemakers and workers,
   (d) people from various ethnic or cultural groups.

5. Summarize and analyze data on your energy balance by including the following:
   (a) Data on body dimensions
      1. Weight and height
      2. Frame size and skin fold
   (b) Data on estimated energy expenditure
      1. Predicted basal metabolism (BMR)
      2. Estimated daily energy expenditure (including BMR)
   (c) Data on dietary intake
      1. Consumption of energy nutrients in diet
      2. Total calories from diet
      3. Percentage calorie distribution in meal pattern
   (d) Analysis coordinating the entire energy expenditure study

APPLICATION OF SKILL IN NUTRITION EDUCATION

From the illustrations given below, design different approaches which can be used to aid people in calorie control to prevent obesity or to correct it.

Too late to eat

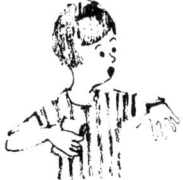

Fig. 6.10 "Too late to eat, so I'll grab a snack."

Group decision

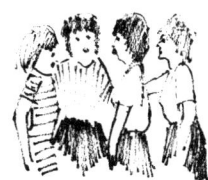

Fig. 6.11 "We all decided to eat lunch at school."

Physical fitness

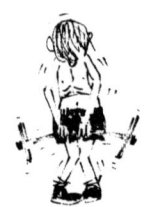

Fig. 6.12 Does physical activity *really* affect calorie balance?

Preaching

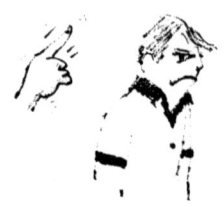

Fig. 6.13 Preaching "good nutrition" does not motivate a teenager to improve his eating habits.

References and Suggested Readings

Abraham, S., and Nordsieck, M. Relationship of excess weight in children and adults, Public Health Rep., **75**, 263 (1960).

Brozek, J. *Human Body Composition.* New York: Pergamon, 1965.

Buskirk, E. R. Problems related to the caloric cost of living, Bulletin, *New York Acad. Med.*, **36**, 63 (1960).

Dwyer, J. T., Feldman, J. J., and Mayer, J. Adolescent dieters, who are they? Physical characteristics, attitudes and dieting practices of adolescent girls, *J. Amer. Dietet. Assoc.*, **56**, 510 (1970).

Eppright, E. S., and Sidwell, V. D. Physical measurements of Iowa school children, *J. Nutr.*, **54**, 543 (1954).

Forbes, G. B. Lean body mass and fat in obese children, *Pediatrics*, **34**, 308 (September 1964).

Forbes, G. B., and Reina, J. C. Adult lean body mass declines with age: Some longitudinal observations, *Metabolism*, **19**, 653 (1970).

Hutson, E. M., Cohen, N. L., Kunkel, N. D., Steinkamp, R. C., Rourke, M. H., and Walsh, H. E. Measures of body fat and related factors in normal adults, *J. Amer. Dietet. Assoc.*, **47**, 179 (1965).

Jacobs, D., Heald, F. P., White, P. L., and McGanity, W. J. Obesity I. Prevention, *J. Amer. Med. Assoc.*, **186**, Suppl., 27 (November 9, 1963).

Keys, A., and Grande, F. Body weight, body composition, and calorie status, Chapter 1 in Wohl and Goodhart's *Modern Nutrition in Health and Disease.* Philadelphia: Lea & Febiger, 1968.

Konishi, F. Food energy equivalents of various activities, *J. Amer. Dietet. Assoc.*, **46**, 186 (1965).

Lamb, M. W., and Michie, J. M. Basal metabolism of nineteen children from two to ten years old, *J. Nutr.*, **53**, 93 (1954).

Mahadeva, K., *et al.* Individual variations in the metabolic cost of standardized exercises; the effects of food, age, sex, and race, *J. Physiol.*, **121**, 225 (1953).

Mayer, J. The physiological basis of obesity and leanness, Part II. *Nutr. Abstr. Rev.*, **25**, 871 (October 1955).

Mayer, J. The role of exercise and activity in weight control, *Weight Control.* Ames, Iowa: Iowa State University Press, 1955.

Personalized Weight Control. Chicago: National Dairy Council, 1966.

Read, M. S., and Heald, F. P. Adolescent obesity—a summary of a symposium, *J. Amer. Dietet. Assoc.*, **47**, 411 (1965).

Seifret, E. The high calorie diet, *Amer. J. Clin. Nutr.*, **12**, 66 (1963).

Seltzer, C. C., Goldman, R. F., and Mayer, J. The triceps skinfold as a predictive measure of body density and body fat in obese adolescent girls, *Pediatrics*, **6**: 2, 212 (August 1965).

Sparge, J. A., Heald, F. P., and Peckos, P. S. Adolescent obesity, *Nutr. Today*, **1**: 4, 4 (1966).

Stefanik, P. A., Heald, F. P., and Mayer, J. Caloric intake in relation to energy output of obese and non-obese adolescent boys, *Amer. J. Clin. Nutr.*, **7**, 55 (January–February 1959).

Stunkard, A., Moore, M. E., and Srole, L. Obesity, social class, and mental illness, *J. Amer. Med. Assoc.*, **181**, 962 (1962).

Swendseid, M. E., Mulcare, D. B., and Drenick, E. J. Nitrogen and weight losses during starvation and realimentation in obesity, *J. Amer. Dietet. Assoc.*, **46**, 276 (April 1965).

Symposium on energy balance, *Amer. J. Clin. Nutr*, **8**, 527 (1960).

The Cell, A scope monograph on cytology. Kalamazoo, Mich.: The Upjohn Co., 1965.

Trulson, M. F., and Stare, F. J. The great balancing act: Eating vs. activity, *Today's Health*, **41**, 35 (1963).

Wright, F. H. Preventing obesity in childhood, *J. Amer. Dietet. Assoc.*, **40**, 516 (1962).

Young, C. M. Some comments on the obesites, *J. Amer. Dietet. Assoc.*, **45**, 134 (1964).

7

Protein as a Source of Amino Acids

Why is Protein Called the Key to Life?

Proteins were referred to as "animal principles" until Beccari in 1728 found them to exist in plants. He separated wheat into an "animal" part (gluten) and a "plant" part (starch). Mulder in 1838 named this "important principle" present in all live matter — protein, which means primary or "holding first place." Even though many nutrients have been identified since then, emphasis on the significance of protein in human welfare is certainly rated paramount in the last of this century.

The role of protein as the key in human nutrition lies in the multiplicity of the protein molecules. Each can consist of all or of some of the 20 amino acids which have been identified in naturally occurring proteins. The number of molecules of amino acids and the sequence in which each occurs determines the protein and its function in a living organism from the unicelled microbe to the complex physiology of man.

Protein is recognized as more than a very complex, high-molecular-weight substance with certain biological value; it is designated by its profile of available amino acids, the units needed to produce enzymes and protoplasm.

Volumes have been written on protein, its sources, regional supplies, conversion by animals into food for people, and its metabolic role in all phases of animal life. Naturally, this section will be a limited presentation on protein as related to people.

THE ROLE OF PROTEIN IN LIFE

Objectives

1. To identify the derivation of amino acids from food and their function in synthesis of proteins in the human body.
2. To distinguish that some amino acids are designated as "nutritionally essential," whereas others can be produced in cells.
3. To recognize the priority system by which the body uses some amino acids for synthesis of one protein in preference to another.

The Sequence of Events Leading to Protein Synthesis

Previously, protein has been identified as one of three classes of organic compounds; proteins differ from carbohydrates and lipids (fats) in that nitrogen is an integral part of each molecule and averages approximately 16% of all natural proteins eaten in a general mixed diet. The nitrogen, a part of every amino acid, occurs as a primary amine group attached to the alpha carbon of certain organic acids.

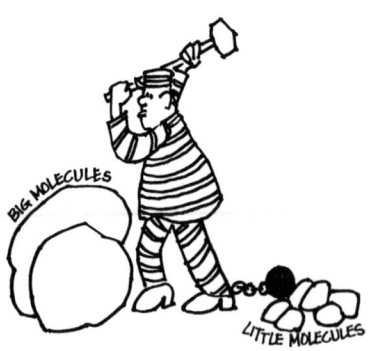

Fig. 7.1 Man has to degradate larger protein molecules into the small ones of amino acids.

The digestive degradation of proteins occurs in the stomach by a proteolytic enzyme which along with proteinases of the duodenal region of the small intestine completes the process producing amino acids available for nutritional processes. The deficient supply of an essential acid from the food protein results in depressed synthesis in the body.

The reaction and structure of amino acids affect their rate of transfer through the intestinal wall into the blood plasma and consequently from plasma to the cell, where they remain free amino acids and provide limited homeostasis. Finally, by this series of complex processes the amino acids enter the capillaries of the villi of the intestinal mucosa, pass then through the portal vein to the liver, and start in the transportation system of the blood to all cells of the body. The liver serves as a limited temporary depot for the amino acids prior to their entering the general blood stream.

Amino acids, combined as peptides and other water soluble proteins, circulate in the blood throughout the body where cells absorb those required for their specific chemical activity. The complexity of the process of absorption through the cell membrane requires several chapters to describe; let it suffice here to recognize that absorption of amino acid compounds is as complex as are the protein substances transported in the blood, 17 of which circulate in the plasma alone. Naturally these proteins are not derived from food only but contain amino acids released by degradation of body proteins from various tissues. The degradation of body proteins occurs at all ages but naturally not at the same rate or to the same degree; furthermore, body conditions of stress including starvation, diseases, infections, and fevers, increase the degradation of body proteins.

Even though the primary need of the body is for energy and protein will contribute to this need upon biological demand, the primary function of protein is synthesis of body proteins needed for life. If a deficit occurs in the energy supply, amino acids will be deaminated at a greater rate than normally and contribute the carbon-hydrogen skeletons to the energy pool. This concept is of increased significance in the current craze for weight control through the use of gross dietary imbalances of the organic classes of nutrients; carbohydrates, fats, and proteins. Especially during childhood this problem is of major concern, since during a period of calorie privation a child would not synthesize sufficient proteins needed for brain, nerve, enzyme, and other development.

Synthesis of protein compounds is directed by the DNA (Deoxyribose Nucleic Acid) in the nucleus through the RNA (Ribose Nucleic Acid) of the ribosomes in the cytoplasm of the cell. However, whether such synthesis occurs in certain cells depends on enzymes and hormones which themselves are composed of amino acids. Some enzymes and hormones cause an increased synthesis in the muscles, others in the liver, and so on; the complete mechanism is not well understood. However, that an intricate interrelationship exists between all nutrients is recognized even if not completely explained.

Synthesis of protein concentrates on the amine and the carboxyl groups of the amino acids as the focal points of their chemical activity. Two amino acids readily combine to form a dipeptide; obviously tri-, tetra-, penta-, and other type peptides can be produced until the amino acid molecules are so numerous that the product is termed a polypeptide and eventually peptones, proteoses and finally, proteins result at the apex of the chemical conglomerate of amino acids with or without other elements or radicals.

$$\underset{\substack{\mid \\ H}}{\overset{\substack{R_1 \\ \mid}}{NH_2-C-COOH}} + \underset{\substack{\mid \\ H}}{\overset{\substack{R_2 \\ \mid}}{NH_2-C-COOH}} + \underset{\substack{\mid \\ H}}{\overset{\substack{R_3 \\ \mid}}{NH_2-C-COOH}}, \text{etc.}$$

R^1, R^2, and R^3 represent the rest of the amino acid molecule which may differ or can be the same amino acid.

The structures of protein molecules are described as a helix in three dimensional space, as a spiral coil of amino acids attached by peptide linkage to each other and occasionally crosslinked with hydrogen and disulfide bonds to stabilize the structure. Plastic and cardboard models of protein molecules are based on actual photographs that have been made by use of the electron microscope. Such pictures support this structural configuration which can be purchased already assembled or in kits for individual creativity. Probably over 100–200 molecules of various amino acids comprise the basic unit of protein structure, which constitute some of the largest molecules synthesized by living organisms.

Proteins cannot be classified simply on the basis of their chemical makeup, since so much remains to be determined about their composition and structure. For this reason the American Society of Biological Chemists and the American Physiological Society classify proteins on the basis of both chemical and physical properties:

1. *Simple proteins* are those which upon hydrolysis yield only amino acids or their derivatives:

   (a) The albumins are soluble in water, coagulated by heat, and usually are low in glycine. They are products of both plants and animals. These proteins include egg albumin, myogen of muscle, serum albumin of blood, lactalbumin of milk, legumelin of peas, and leucosin of wheat.

   (b) *Globulins* generally contain the nonessential amino acid, glycine, are insoluble in water and are heat coagulable such as ovoglobulin of egg yolk, serum globulin of blood, myosin of muscle, edestin of hemp seed, phaseolin of beans, legumin of peas, excelsin of Brazil nuts, arachin of peanuts, and amandin of almonds.

   (c) *Glutelins* are soluble in very dilute acids and alkalies, are insoluble in neutral solvents and are plant proteins such as glutenin of wheat and oryzenin of rice.

(d) *Prolamins* are alcohol-soluble proteins which usually contain proline and amide nitrogen but are deficient in lysine such as zein of corn, hordein of barley, gliadin of wheat, and kafirin of kafir corn.

(e) *Albuminoids* or scleroproteins are the least soluble of all proteins. These are animal proteins only and are the chief constituents of exoskeletal structures such as hair, horn, hoofs, and nails, as well as fibrous tissues and the organic material of cartilage and bone. Examples include keratins of hair, horn, hoofs, nails; elastin of connective tissue; collagen of bones, cartilage and tendons; spongin of sponges; and fibroin and sericin of silk.

(f) *Histones*, being basic proteins usually occur in salt combinations with acidic substances such as heme of hemoglobin and nucleic acids. Examples include globin of hemoglobin, thymus histones, scombrone of mackerel sperm, etc.

(g) *Protamins* are the simplest of the proteins and may be regarded as large polypeptides; like the histones they usually occur in tissues in salt combination with acids, for example, combined with nucleic acids as nucleoproteins of sperm.

2. *Conjugated proteins* are composed of a simple protein combined with a nonprotein substance referred to as a prosthetic (addition) group:

(a) Nucleoproteins are simple basic proteins (protamines or histones) combined with nucleic acids and are abundant in both plant and animal tissues. They are the proteins of cell nuclei and examples are nucleohistone and nucleoprotamin.

(b) Mucoproteins are composed of simple proteins combined with mucopolysaccharides such as hyaluronic acid and the chrondroitin sulfates. They are usually present in all kinds of animal mucins and in the blood group substances.

(c) Chromoproteins are composed of simple proteins combined with a colored prosthetic group such as hemoglobins, cytochromes, flavoproteins, melanin (the pigment of skin and hair), and others. Visual purple of the retina is a chromoprotein in which a carotenoid pigment is the prosthetic group.

(d) Phosphoproteins such as the casein of milk and vitellin of egg yolk are combinations of simple proteins and phosphoric acid as the prosthetic group.

(e) Lipoproteins are composed of simple proteins combined with a lipid such as lecithin, cephalin, some fatty acid, etc. These occur in milk, blood, egg yolk, cell membranes, etc.

(f) Metalloproteins are a large group of enzyme proteins which contain metallic elements such as iron, copper, cobalt, manganese, and others as the prosthetic group. Heme proteins are also metalloproteins, as well as chromoproteins.

3. *Derived proteins* are formed by hydrolytic cleavage of peptide bonds in simple and conjugated proteins and may be considered either as primary or secondary derived proteins.

(a) Primary derived proteins are the denatured protein which includes proteans such as fibrin from fibrinogen in blood clot formation; metaproteins as acid and alkaline albuminates, and coagulated proteins such as albumin in cooked egg and in cooked meat, etc.

(b) Secondary derived proteins are from large protein molecules and can be grouped into proteoses, peptones, and peptides.

(c) The stepwise degradation of the protein molecule into derived products is given in this sequence:

protein → protean → metaprotein → proteose → peptone → → peptides → amino acids

This brief summary of classes of proteins gives an overview of the complexity of proteins in human tissues. It indicates combinations of other molecules with amino acids to form complex specialized molecules. Products derived from proteins represent both hydrolysis which occurs during digestion and degradation of the molecule in cellular catabolism.

Amino acids, too, represent a variety of molecular structures with each containing an alpha amino carboxylic group. They are classified on the basis of chemical structure and activity:

1. The number of amino and carboxyl groups present in the molecule, such as monoaminomonocarboxylic acids and monoaminodicarboxylic acids, etc.

2. Aliphatic, aromatic, and heterocyclic amino acids are grouped according to the presence of the type of carbon chain and ring structures.

3. Their reaction in solutions as neutral, acidic, and basic amino acids.

4. Their roles in animal nutrition dependent on dietary supply of selected ones in preformation of molecules.

Table 7.1   Classification of amino acids.

Essential (need to be supplied as formed molecules)	Nonessential (can be synthesized from cellular substances)
Lysine	Glycine
Tryptophan	Alanine
Phenylalanine	Serine
Leucine	Cystine
Isoleucine	Tyrosine
Threonine	Aspartic Acid
Methionine	Glutamic Acid
Valine	Proline
Histidine*	Citrulline
Arginine*	Hydroxyproline

*Essential only for the growing child.

CLASSIFICATION OF NUTRITIONALLY ESSENTIAL AMINO ACIDS

A. Aliphatic amino acids with carbon chain structure:
   1. Monoaminomonocarboxylic acids are *neutral* in reaction.
      Example: threonine, alpha-amino-beta-hydroxy-*n*-butyric acid

$$CH_3-CHOH-CH-COOH$$
$$|$$
$$NH_2$$

Other amino acids of this class and their chemical name based on the configuration involved are:
Methionine, alpha-amino-gama-methylthio-*n*-butyric acid
Leucine, alpha-amino-isocaproic acid
Isoleucine, alpha-amino-beta-methyl-*n*-valeric acid
Valine, alpha-amino-isovaleric acid
   2. Diaminomonocarboxylic acids are *basic* in chemical activity:
      Example: lysine, alpha-epsilon-di-amino-*n*-caproic acid

$$NH_2-CH_2-CH_2-CH_2-CH_2-CH-COOH$$
$$|$$
$$NH_2$$

   Arginine is another amino acid in this class, delta-guanidine-amino-valeric acid
B. Aromatic amino acids are monoaminomonocarboxylic and *neutral* in reaction:
   Example: phenylalanine, alpha-amino-beta-phenyl-propionic acid

$$C_6H_5-CH_2-CH-COOH$$
$$|$$
$$NH_2$$

C. Heterocyclic amino acids are monoaminomonocarboxylic acids and *neutral* in reaction except histidine which is *slightly basic*:

Example: histidine, alpha-amino-beta-imidazole-propionic acid

$$HC\!\!=\!\!\!=\!\!\!=\!\!C\!-\!CH_2\!-\!CH\!-\!COOH$$

$$\begin{array}{ccc} | & | & | \\ N & NH & NH_2 \\ \diagdown & \diagup & \\ & CH & \end{array}$$

Tryptophan is another amino acid in this class, alpha-amino-beta-indole-propionic acid.

The nonessential amino acids can be classified under these divisions and are included in organic chemistry books.

The Cell as the Center of Synthesis and Life

General description of protein synthesis appears as though it were a hodgepodge of activity; actually, each individual cell directs synthesis in a highly systematic order. A muscle cell carries the design for all proteins which constitute its structure or that are required to reproduce another cell of identical properties. Its identification has been traced to a system of coded directions in the complex deoxyribose nucleic acid (DNA) in the cell nucleus which in turn releases smaller ribose nucleic acids (RNA). These migrate from the nucleus into the cytoplasm of the cell to become attached to ribosomes. The RNA directs the sequence of amino acids that are required for the specific protein involved. One hypothesis specifies that one RNA molecule serves as a model or template on which amino acids are aligned in the order specified, while another RNA molecule may assemble amino acids from the "nutrient pool" in the cell and furnish the amino acid to the ribosome in the position it needs to occupy in the new protein. Apparently, specific enzymes are produced simultaneously to activate the proper amino acid for chemical activity at its designated place in the new chain.

Naturally, each protein has its own particular sequence of amino acids as directed by the DNA code. An amino acid must be activated to form the high energy peptide bond between the acid group and the amino group of another acid. The energy is derived from adenosine triphosphate (ATP), the energy releasing mechanism of every living cell.

Each pair of amino acids to be linked up and "hooked" together requires a separate mechanism which the RNA transfers to the site of synthesis of the new protein molecule. As many mechanisms exist as are required for the peptide linkages. The newly produced protein molecule then migrates to its position in the cell or tissue to replace old fragmented molecules that were to be replaced. The cell constantly synthesizes new molecules to replace others or to increase the total quantity (growth); the rate and duration of such activity depends on the tissue and its general metabolism in the person involved, his age, health, and overall activity pattern. Naturally, if the supply of amino acids required for synthesis lacks one or has an imbalance in the supply for the assortment required, synthesis cannot occur unless the deficit is corrected promptly. No evidence indicates a "holding action" during a delay of protein synthesis.

The living cell is a site of constant chemical change; when synthesis or anabolism exceeds degradation or catabolism in the cell or tissue, then increase in number and/or mass of that type of cell should occur and the individual tissue grows. On the other hand, if the reverse is true, then the quantity of tissue is reduced and the person may deteriorate in physical well-being proportionately. An assumption is that in the adult at the prime of life the two processes are equal and little change occurs in body composition. Obviously, synthesis depends on the supply of amino acids available at all times to the cells as well as on the other nutritional factors required.

Proteins in Body Function

A unique angle to protein synthesis is that an adequate supply of certain amino acids has to be furnished as molecules by the general supply of protein in the diet. In the early years of search for optimum diets, those proteins which promoted normal growth when fed in certain amounts in otherwise adequate diets were referred to as "complete proteins;" those that failed to do so were designated as "incomplete proteins." In this early animal feeding research, both the specific protein and its level in the diet were proved to be involved. Thus a complete protein was identified as "partially complete" when the ratio in the diet was suboptimal, e.g., at levels of casein below 18–24% of the dry weight for rats. The fact is that differences in the nutritional quality of proteins are more accurately stated as differences in the ability of dietary proteins to support normal protein synthesis in a test animal. Such differences are attributed to the quantity of the essential amino acids of each protein; at first only the assortment of amino acids was considered but eventually with refined chemical analytical methods and equipment, the quantity required of each "essential amino acid" was identified. These "nutrionally essential amino acids" are really inaccurately named; the term refers to their preformation by either plant or other animals prior to ingestion by a person. They should be termed "dietetically essential" in that these molecules must be supplied by the diet. The other amino acids which can be synthesized by the human body are also nutritionally essential but the molecules themselves do not need to be furnished by the diet.

Undoubtedly, the emphasis on growth and protein has encouraged some affluent, eager and overzealous parents to overfeed their children with supplies of amino acids to a point that physical maturity is attained at younger years. The idea has been dramatically stated that overnutrition with high quality protein "has put sex into the hands of children" or "has produced fully grown mature bodies with immature minds and social behavior." The question is constantly raised, "Is the goal of adequate nutrition to raise giants in the least number of years?" Such results have been achieved by agriculture in production of poultry, swine, and cattle; e.g., a two-pound broiler in six weeks, a 200-pound pig in six months, or a 1000-pound beef in less than two years. Edible meat production is a goal which should be considerably different from that of human development where emphasis is on performance and longevity. This is a concern in the world as a whole and of people within an affluent nation since it takes much more food, space, and environment to support giant bodies than smaller ones.

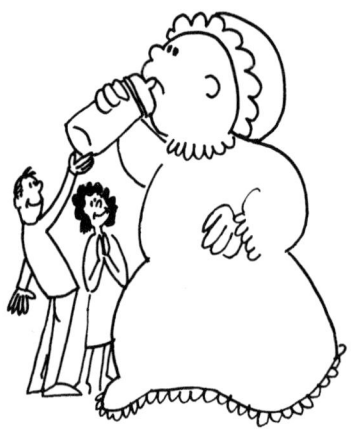

Fig. 7.2   Is the goal of nutrition to raise giants?

The protein supply within a hen's egg has been proved to contain the best ratio of amounts of all nutritionally essential amino acids for growth of children as well as chicks. The Food and Agriculture Organization (FAO) of the United Nations has attempted to replicate this assortment as shown in Table 7.3, p. 180. Such proportions are often referred to as amino acid patterns: the Egg Pattern or FAO Amino Acid Pattern. These patterns serve as guides for chemical evaluation of a protein or of mixtures of protein as eaten in a daily dietary regimen. Obviously such an assortment of amino acids would function only within a supply sufficient in total protein and a diet adequate in energy from carbohydrate and fats, and in mineral elements and vitamins.

A person should keep in mind that relatively little is known about protein synthesis in any specific type cell in the human body. Most hypotheses about pathways of protein synthesis refer to the hypothetical, *typical cell*. One can only speculate as to how the processes differ in a muscle cell from a nerve cell, a brain cell, or a bone cell. Every cell has its pattern of protein synthesis. Furthermore, what is the priority system within the human body? If an essential amino acid is supplied at a 50% level of sufficiency, which tissue cells will have enough, which will be deprived, or do all tissue cells share equally in the suboptimal supply of the required amino acid? Perhaps, even a natural priority system functions during the period of development of a child which determines the tissue priority for protein synthesis; e.g., at age two, synthesis of brain tissue proteins undoubtedly have preference over the proteins in muscle cells since at this age brain matures more rapidly than skeletal muscle.

Certain failures in protein synthesis have been reported in women on highly restricted reducing diets who ceased to menstruate until dietary intakes were more liberal or better balanced. Infants of normal growth when weaned from a regular feeding schedule grow at less than average increments, show stunting in size, and retardation in development as compared to averages of adequately fed infants.

Even the incomplete knowledge of today supports the fact that protein synthesis in all cells is crucial to the health of a person at any age and under any condition. Thus the role of a regular supply of preformed amino acids with enough total protein in an adequate diet greatly enhances the well-being of people.

Activities for Student Learning

1. Study the stages of child development in order to identify the tissues undergoing the most rapid maturation and thereby speculate on the priority for protein synthesis.
2. Relate the structure of the protein molecule to the properties of proteins as seen in food proteins; envision the degradation of the huge complex protein molecule through the different stages to polypeptides and finally to the individual amino acids.
3. Study research on protein restriction in laboratory or domestic animals, noting the influence on growth caused by such variations as in quantity of protein in the adequate diet; e.g., 20% casein in contrast to a 10% level, or the source of protein in the diet such as egg proteins in contrast to corn proteins or casein in contrast to zein, or amino acid supplementation of an "incomplete protein."

DIETARY NEED FOR AMINO ACIDS (PROTEIN)

Objectives

1. To be aware of the principles of procedures used to establish physiological use and need for protein.
2. To recognize conditions in people which affect the need and utilization of protein for tissue synthesis and maintenance.
3. To be able to plan for energy deficits without seriously affecting protein synthesis in adults.
4. To identify periods and conditions of stress that affect dietary intake, digestion, and protein synthesis in people.
5. To understand the protein requirements that are specified by a dietary regimen.

Methods to Determine Protein Requirements

The Law of Conservation of Energy and Mass, neither energy nor matter is created or destroyed but may change form, applies to the living organism. Thus all the food consumed by a person is processed and disposed of in some way. In general, certain steps that are involved in assessing the quality of dietary protein include:

(a) A period of several days in which to establish the dietary pattern of the person or experimental animal.
(b) The determination of the protein content of food eaten through nitrogen analysis. Since proteins in general consist of a mean nitrogen content of 16%, a factor 6.25 times the grams of nitrogen is equivalent to grams of protein. Usually a representative sample (an aliquot) of 1–5% of the weight of each dietary component is collected at each meal and snack; these are combined to represent the total day's food intake. This can be considered *gross nitrogen intake*.
(c) During the test or experimental period, feces are collected and analyzed for nitrogen content. Feces contain undigested dietary protein and proteins from digestive secretions and mucous from the walls of the gastrointestinal tract. Even though these proteins are both from exogenous and endogenous sources, for a subject under controlled conditions, the endogenous nitrogen loss is constant. The nitrogen content of the feces is deducted from that in the diet giving the quantity of *net nitrogen intake*.
(d) Urinary excretion is also collected and analyzed for total nitrogen, the amount of urea, and other nitrogenous compounds. Urea

represents the nitrogen removed from amino acids by deamination and includes both exogenous and endogenous amino acids. Urinary nitrogen is of metabolic origin and represents the excreta from cellular life. A comparison of this quantity of nitrogen with the net nitrogen intake will designate the nitrogen balance for that day or experimental period.

Naturally, some daily variation in nitrogen balance occurs in normal people, nonetheless certain generalizations can be made:

1. If the net nitrogen intake equaled the urinary excretion, the individual is in *zero nitrogen balance*; the intake was sufficient to meet the output. Neither addition to the quantity of body protein nor loss occurred. This does not mean that nothing happened, but that anabolic processes had enough supplies to meet catabolic ones in order to maintain the *status quo* of the tissues of the body.

2. If the net nitrogen intake exceeded the excretion, nitrogen-containing molecules were retained and the body was in *positive nitrogen balance*. In this case, an increase in protein-tissue mass occurred or the protein was excreted in milk, lost in hemorrhage, or by other means. Such a balance must occur for growth in childhood or pregnancy, during lactation, in recovery from a wasting disease (one in which tissue mass was reduced), and in some cases of athletic training in which muscle mass increased.

3. The last type of balance to occur is called *negative nitrogen balance* in that net nitrogen intake is less than urinary excretion resulting in a decrease of protein in the body. Such a condition results from deficient amount or poor quality of dietary protein intake and also from calorie deficient or reducing diets. Any diet or condition which causes decrease in mass of body tissues, even adipose tissue, causes increased urinary nitrogen excretion which, if not offset by increased dietary intake, will develop into a negative nitrogen balance. In addition to deficits in the diet, infections, fevers, hemorrhages, diarrhea (which includes increased mucous excretion) and other physiological disturbances cause such an increased nitrogen excretion and body tissue loss.

Obviously, when a child does not grow during negative nitrogen balance, he would be retarded in development, maturation or growth. Recovery would be possible in proportion to the severity and duration of the negative balance as well as the age or developmental stage of the child. Even though negative balance fluctuates and a zero balance will result from different levels of protein intake, it is a valuable tool by which to assess protein requirements of a person as well as to determine the biological value of a diet.

Influences on Protein Requirements

From the description of results obtained in balance studies, the manipulation of the dietary supply of nutrients proved to be a major factor in achieving the desired nitrogen balance. However, the supply of nutrients is only significant in the framework of the need of the human body and its utilization of the nutrients. For example, a so-called "average or normal child" would be in positive nitrogen balance on a diet with 1.4 g of protein per kilogram body weight and at 2200 calories intake; another child of the same age range who is in a more rapid than average rate of growth or who is hyperactive in physical activity may be in zero or even negative nitrogen balance on the same dietary intake. Generalizations are acceptable only as long as the individual person is not overlooked and adjustments are made for his needs.

Characteristics which affect the nitrogen balance and thereby the protein and energy needs of an individual are multiple:

1. Age influences the dietary needs as related to individual rates of growth and maturation and to adult maintenance.
2. Pregnancy and lactation are periods of stress which demand nutrient supplies for tissue building and for secretion of milk in addition to normal body functions. The amount of milk secretion is proportionate to the adequacy of the diet and especially to that of protein.
3. Energy expenditure reflects both basal metabolism and energy required in muscular exertion. In order to minimize the use of amino acids as sources of energy, sufficient carbohydrates and fats must be supplied to avoid negative nitrogen balance. The greater the calorie deficit, the greater the nitrogen loss. For example, on reducing diets of 900 calories or less, the body tissue loss is about 60% protoplasm, whereas on 1200 calories and higher levels of calorie intake, only about 40% of the body loss is calculated to be protoplasm. Obviously, children cannot grow on a calorie deficient diet.

   Muscular performance does not increase catabolism of protein so that neither athletes, laborers, nor sportsmen require a larger amount of protein but the same ratio of carbohydrate, fat, and protein as sedentary individuals. This assumes that no increase in muscularity or recovery from emaciation occurs such as implied in training or in recovery when a higher dietary intake is required to produce a positive nitrogen balance. During game competitition when athletic directors gorge their players on meat, milk, cheese, and eggs, they do so for the status prestige of such foods. In fact, the athlete may be handicapped by a high protein intake which places a stress on the liver and kidneys for deamination and excretion of urea and other nitrogen compounds.

4. Certain physiological conditions affect digestion, absorption, and tissue need for protein. For example, digestive efficiency and percentage of absorption of ingested nutrients remains an individual characteristic and may be an asset or a detriment to food efficiency. The motility of the contents of the digestive tract can affect digestion and subsequent absorption of nutrients. The role of diarrhea in contributing to negative nitrogen balance has been established. Also, the influence of dietary composition is significant, especially in young children and in aged people. For example, diets high either in sugar, fat, or cellulose can interfere with digestion and absorption of nutrients. Some physiologists have postulated that people with short stature have a lower motility rate and higher absorption of nutrients which contributes to the ease of obesity in contrast to those who are tall of linear build and "never gain a pound" even though they eat heartily.

Diseases involving fevers increase the rate of catabolism of protein and of cells in addition to the energy cost both for the fever itself (7% increase in BMR per degree Fahrenheit of fever) and for activity associated with restlessness. Debilitating diseases including malignancies and other degenerative anomalies require increased proteins in an effort to refurnish wasting tissues.

Metabolic disturbances involving enzyme and hormone inbalances may change protein metabolism although little is known or understood about these conditions in the early stages of growth.

5. Varying degrees of starvation, whether due to food shortage, improper food for age, imbalance of nutrients, parasites, anorexia, voluntary dietary eccentricities, self-chosen faddism, or to any combination of these, all of these affect nitrogen balance unfavorably. Whenever the period of dietary privation has been long or the extent severe, the individual may have had loss of digestive enzyme production or of the mucosal wall to make absorption almost impossible. Parenteral feeding is often indicated until recovery allows for readily digestible foods to be eaten. Most recent developments indicate that feeding directly into the *vena cava*

avoids some of the disadvantages of intravenous feeding into veins near the surface as in the arm or hand.

6. Theories derived from research on the aging process indicate that the chronic dietary supplies of certain nutrients may play a crucial role in maintenance of the prime of life. After 65 years, even an increased amount of protein may be needed. Data on laboratory animals support the theories and indicate that the sulfur-containing amino acids (methionine and cystine) are among the several nutrients implicated, according to Passwater and Welker in a 1971 review. The time has come not to add years of senility but to add years of useful living to the human life-span.

7. Physical anomalies such as those in cerebral palsied children have unknown demands on the nutrients supplied to these individuals. Almost nothing is known about the needs and benefits to be derived from various levels of nutrient intake of handicapped children and adults. Since handicaps that persons have often involve eating and reduce their ability to feed themselves, their diets have been very uncertain. These children are often kept on limited and monotonous diets; they are indulged in their natural acceptance of sweets which contributes to excess weight and difficulty in handling the handicapped person. A nutritionally balanced high quality protein and adequate calorie intake should certainly be considered essential for handicapped persons.

8. Environmental stress such as cold may cause increased nitrogen excretion and subsequently higher dietary intakes. Long-term research is urgently needed to study the dietary needs of individuals migrating to Arctic and Antarctic areas on military bases or oil and mineral industry projects.

Biological Value of Food Proteins

The biological value (BV) of a protein is an expression of a number of the nutritional characteristics of the food. These include (1) the digestibility, (2) the availability of the digested products, and (3) the presence and amounts of the various essential amino acids. The biological value can be calculated by determining the nitrogen of the food intake minus the urinary and fecal nitrogen excretions by the formula:

$$BV = \frac{\text{Dietary N} - (\text{Urinary N} + \text{Fecal N})}{\text{Dietary N} - \text{Fecal N}} \times 100.$$

The biological value of some proteins fed either to rats or humans is given in Table 7.2. The biological values reported in the literature for some of the proteins by different researchers vary in numerical value, suggesting that as yet, no definite assessment can be made. When 70% of the intake of nitrogen is retained (a biological value of 70) the protein will support growth if sufficient calories are available; with biological values of less than 70, questionable growth occurs.

Table 7.2 Comparison of the biological value of selected proteins.

Food	Bases for biological value	
	Human adult	Growing rat
Egg	94, 97	87
Milk	62, 79, 100	90
Fish	94	75
Beef muscle	67, 75, 80, 84	76
White flour	42, 40, 67, 70	52
Soy flour	65, 71, 81	75
Navy bean	46	38

Concurrently catabolism and anabolism of protein are occurring in the body; for anabolism to operate efficiently, all of the essential amino acids must be available in the sufficient quantity. If they are not, excess nitrogen is excreted in the urine due to the catabolic process. When this occurs, less absorbed food nitrogen is retained by the body and low biological value results from feeding this protein or protein mixture.

The biological value of soybean proteins is improved by heat treatment, probably due to methionine becoming more readily available to the organism. In the untreated soybeans the release of methionine seems to be delayed so that absorption occurs too late in the intestinal transit. For optimum utilization of protein all the essential amino acids must be liberated during digestion at rates allowing mutual supplementation.

If a high biological value protein contains a balance of amino acids in the proportion required by the body, then probably an excessive addition of one or more amino acids can cause an imbalance. No adequate explanation for the imbalance phenomenon is available but this idea dictates the theory that amino acids should not be added to food indiscriminately. Advocates of lysine supplementation of bread may be premature in their promotion.

Net protein utilization (NPU) is another index which combines a measure of the biological value and the digestibility of the protein in a diet. For a given diet, NPU is determined by calculations from chemical score data:

$$NPU = \frac{biological\ value \times digestibility}{N\ retained/N\ intake}.$$

Net protein utilization is determined under standard conditions at a fixed level of protein intake below maintenance and is a practical method of evaluating differences in protein quality.

Other animal assay technics may be used to determine the biological value of protein. These technics and technical terms are described in the National Academy of Science – National Research Council Publication, *Evaluation of Protein Quality*.

Protein efficiency ratio. Protein efficiency ratio (PER) is the easiest method of assessing the quality of proteins. Generally accepted is the idea that the rate of growth of weanling rats under standardized conditions provides a reliable measure of the value of dietary protein; thus PER is the gain in body weight divided by the amount of protein consumed:

$$PER = \frac{weight\ gain}{protein\ intake}.$$

Such factors as the age of the rats, length of the experimental period, level of protein, and the sex of the rat affect the PER assay. Optimum standardized conditions such as a four-week experimental feeding period, diets containing a 10% level of protein with sufficient amounts of all other essential nutrients, male rats, and *ad libitum* feeding schedule have been demonstrated by several laboratories to yield reproducible results.

The PER determination has been criticized on the basis that (1) gain in body weight may not be constant in tissue composition on diets containing different proteins, (2) results may vary with protein level, and (3) the determination makes no allowance for the maintenance requirement.

Analysis of foods for amino acid content. Current developments of relatively simple methods for quantitative determination of the amino acids in protein hydrolyzates prepared from foods, such as the microbiological, enzymatic, and chromatographic methods, have made available a "chemical scoring" of protein. This scoring is based on the assumption that the nutritive value of protein is dependent upon the amino acid composition; i.e., the protein is as good as its combination of the essential amino acids.

The Food and Agriculture Organization has established provisional patterns for the essential amino acids based on the minimum amino acid requirements determined experimentally with young adults fed purified amino acid diets. This pattern, as well as the pattern of egg protein, has been used as a reference standard and is shown in Table 7.4, p. 181. Additional experimental studies are needed for further interpretation of the effectiveness of the combinations of amino acids suggested by these patterns.

Many common foods have been analyzed for their essential amino acid content and these results have been reported by M. L. Orr and B. K. Watt of the USDA. Thus, a guide for designing nutritionally satisfactory meals containing proteins of different origins and chemical scores is available. The chemical evaluation of protein agrees with some of the values obtained by the more complicated biological methods. But in many cases, the actual biological value is lower than that predicted on the basis of the amino acid composition because not all of the amino acids present in food are physiologically available; utilization depends on the nature of the B_3 linkages by which they are connected within the protein molecule. If such linkages are not hydrolyzed by the particular enzyme that is present, the amino acids involved are not liberated and may be lost with the feces or destroyed by the intestinal flora.

Supplementary value of proteins. The supplementary action of one food protein to another is of special interest, since rarely does a human being or an animal consume a single protein in his pattern of eating. When two proteins are fed together, the biological value is greater than when either protein is fed alone and higher than the calculated average value would indicate. For example, if one protein had a biological value of 70 and another of 50, and these were combined in a 50-50 ratio in a diet, the value would be expected to be 60. Instead, it may be 67 or even 80 if the amino acid concentrations "match," which means that one protein had a generous supply of the amino acid present in only deficit amounts in the other protein. To illustrate, gelatin is an incomplete protein since it lacks tryptophan and has a very limited amount of several other essential amino acids but it has a relatively high concentration of lysine. On the other hand, wheat gluten is low in lysine and higher in tryptophan, methionine, and others. Gelatin and wheat gluten combined produced better growth than either fed alone. Other examples include the proteins of beans and peas which lacking in the sulfur-containing amino acids contain sufficient amounts of lysine, and have considerable supplementary value when added to cereals in a diet. Other food combinations to show supplementary protein value are peanut butter and milk, rice and fish, etc.

Protein Undernutrition

Even though protein foods are plentiful in the United States, deficiencies of dietary protein exist which result in stunted growth and poor development. Such data were reported in the recent nutrition survey (Schaefer, 1969) made in several states of the United States.

Dietary studies in the United States have identified certain groups of people to be the most vulnerable targets for protein undernutrition. These groups are the low income and welfare families whose income and assistance is low, their knowledge is insufficient to supply adequate food, and their management ability is undeveloped. Such families often have a woman as head who is untrained for employment and is restricted by child care responsibilities. They often live in environments which increase health risks and cost of survival. Another target group centers on school children, especially those in deprived urban areas. Probably a universal school lunch program will soon function which requires no payment from the children or the parents and will be dominantly tax supported.

Another target group in the United States is the aged, predominantly the single men and women living alone whose spouse has already died. These people have very limited facilities to shop for food, to prepare food, and worst of all is the loss of incentive to want to continue to try. The "meals on wheels" program and other community centered programs are being tried to determine acceptance, cost, and efficiency. Publications of reports of the many studies and surveys can be found in professional and lay literature.

World nutrition and the problems of protein–calorie malnutrition are now included in most nutrition textbooks. Numerous publications from FAO, WHO, and agencies of the United States as well as other organizations give data about many populations in the world. Numerous syndromes of hunger such as edema, pellagra, kwashiorkor, marasmus, mental retardation, lowered resistance to diseases, and other are associated with one or multiple dietary deficiencies.

Organizations of the United Nations and other international and regional agencies are concerned with the nutrition of the people of the world and are endeavoring to close the gaps between food eaten, protein needs, protein quality and supply, and efficiency of energy intake. Lowenberg, *et al.* (1968) presented a very good discussion of these international and national programs and their efforts to relieve hunger and malnutrition. Increasing recognition and emphases are placed on food habits, customs, cultures, and religion as causative factors as well as avenues of approach to solutions. Anthropologists, sociologists, phychologists, and other social scientists as well as nutritionists are recognizing food and eating to be more than satisfying hunger, that people do not eat "because it is good for them to do so," that food aversions can serve as a measurement of psychosis, and that nutrition involves all segments of society.

Anomalies of Amino Acid Metabolism

No living matter, as yet identified, is devoid of protein. Proteins, or amino acids, in combination with nucleic acids carry the inheritance factors (DNA and RNA) for the individual; small alterations in the structure of the nucleoproteins of cells may lead to disease or aberrant physical development. Some 70 inborn errors of metabolism in infants and children have been recognized; for most of these, appropriate nutritional therapy is of some value to further the normal development of the child if the condition was identified early and therapy followed. The following list describes some of the most frequently diagnosed conditions:

> *Celiac disease* is a chronic intestinal disorder of infants and young children characterized by intolerance of raw milk protein and wheat or rye gluten.
>
> *Cystinuria* causes a loss of amino acid, cystine, in the urine because of renal tubular disorders and may cause kidney stones; it requires dietary manipulation of fluids and condiments.
>
> *Histidinemia* caused by an absence of the enzyme histidase, can result in a speech defect.
>
> *Maple sugar urine disease* which was named for the characteristic odor, is due to a block in the oxidative decarboxylation of the branched chain amino acids. Early diagnosis and dietary regulation may result in some amelioration of the disease.
>
> *Phenylketonuria* is a hereditary disorder in protein metabolism in which phenylalanine is not metabolized to tyrosine because of enzyme deficiency, and its intermediate products are excreted in the urine. The result can be severe mental impairment, loss of pigment in skin, hair, and eyes, a cessation of growth, development, and inability to speak depending on the extent of deficiency of the enzyme.

Most persons with phenylketonuria (PKU) are the offspring of two heterozygous carriers of the defective gene, who may also have normal children. The incidence of PKU is one in every 10,000 births, so it may be calculated that one person in 50 is a carrier for this disorder. Many, but not all, states in the United States have passed laws to test newborn infants for PKU. Previously the test used for detection was the reaction that resulted in a characteristic dark green-blue color reaction when ferric chloride was added to urine in a wet diaper. A newer method, the Guthrie test, is based on testing the blood of infants 24 or more hours after the onset of milk feeding and has proved to be more satisfactory.

Clinical experience indicates that if control with a low phenylalanine diet is instituted early in infancy, a good chance exists to prevent mental deficiency. Once brain development has become retarded, the process can only be arrested, not reversed. Experience with dietary management is still new.

A certain amount of phenylalanine (15–30 mg/kg or 7–14 mg/lb) is needed for normal growth and development; individual dietary management is required because of variation between patients. Urine and blood levels of phenylalanine, progress in growth and mental development, and prevention or relief of mental and physical symptoms serve as guides for dietary planning. New developments in treatment are constantly being reported.

Protein Requirements Met by Menu Design

To define minimum protein requirements for healthy normal or average people is limited by the adequacy of the technics used. Studies on protein requirements are based on three approaches depending on whether the dietary supply or the person's response to a protein of known quality is to be tested:

1. determination of amount of essential amino acids required to maintain nitrogen balance,
2. determination of total amount of protein required for nitrogen balance, and
3. estimation of nitrogen losses that have to be met in the dietary supply of protein.

Studies to determine protein requirements usually concentrate on the average reference man or child. A protein that is considered to be completely utilized is chosen and the diet is planned to maintain a fixed adequate calorie intake. Naturally, some variations occur in the results. FAO–WHO has proposed these estimates required by the average reference man and child:

Reference Person	*g protein/kg body weight*
Average adult	0.59
One to three-year-old child	0.88
Newborn to three-month-old infant	2.30

Since the RDA includes a "margin for safety," the amounts of protein recommended in an average mixed diet are adequate and not minimum as noted in Fig. 7.3.

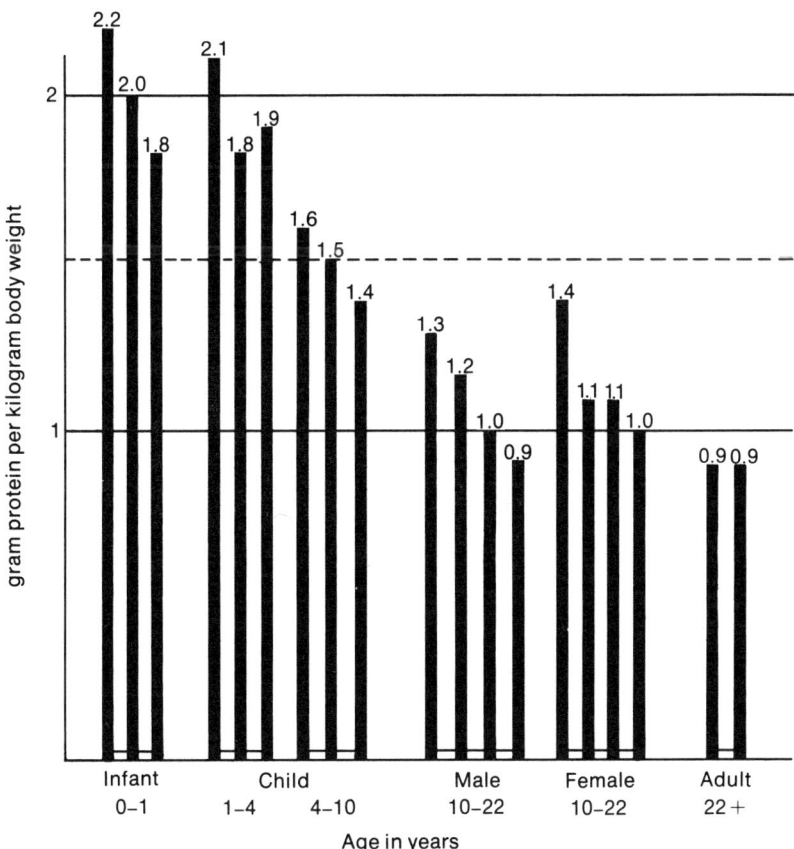

Fig. 7.3 Recommended protein per kilogram of weight at age intervals (NRC's 1968 revision).

The high protein needs during childhood parallel the energy needs so that the traditional allowance of 10–15% of the calories derived from protein allows a sufficient amino acid supply for growth in children. However, one can note quickly the detrimental effect of consuming foods which supply mostly carbohydrate and fat and not the prescribed amount of protein. Since children often eat only one or two foods at a time, the so-called "empty calorie" meals can damage development and retard the growth pattern. Research on domestic animals has shown the advantage of pelletized balanced rations in which each bite has a balance in nutrient content. Contrast the results of such balanced eating to one in which a preschool child eats high carbohydrate and fat "goodies," such as this sample menu:

A SAMPLE MENU

At breakfast (4 g protein)	3 oz fruit or juice 1 average pancake with butter and syrup 1 sl. bacon
At lunch (4 g protein)	½ C chicken-noodle soup with 2 crackers ½ apple (fruits or melons) 2 plain cookies
Snacktime	6 oz popular sweetened or artificially sweetened drinks, either liquid or frozen on a stick
Evening meal (6 g protein)	meat (mostly rejected since it was not adapted to the chewing capacity of the teeth at this age) ½ C nonseed type vegetables 1 sl. bread ⅛ sector 2 crust fruit pie iced tea

Total protein intake 14 g; 25–30 g is recommended intake.

Perhaps few preschool children eat such an assortment of calorie supply, but some do whenever the mother or whoever supervises the dietary intake follows an unplanned, haphazard feeding or eating schedule. Stress on quality protein intake at regular intervals for young children cannot be overemphasized. The development of the superego, reduced rate of growth, decreased appetite with reduced activity, the lack of molar teeth for chewing, and some teeth that loosen and shed leaving gaps and tender sore gums, all these complicate the eating pattern and food acceptance of the preschool child from three to six years old. The older school child usually has developed a taste for protein foods and can manipulate eating and chewing them. Also, as the energy needs of the active older

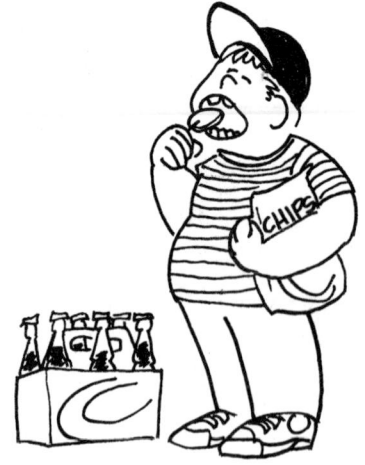

Fig. 7.4 The "empty calorie" foods can damage development.

child increase, his appetite increases and he gets a wider variety of foods contributing to the protein supply in his diet.

In planning family meals, a source of high quality protein should be included each time food is served whether it is a major meal or only a snack. Children can enhance their intake of lower quality or quantity of protein food by drinking milk either with a meal or with a snack in order that a pint to a quart of milk is consumed daily and adequate protein is supplied at each eating time. The mother, on the other hand, has the opportunity and the responsibility to incorporate sufficient protein into the foods which the child will eat. She really needs to acquire the concept "to prepare foods with a purpose"; she can increase the protein content of many foods prepared at home or even of those bought as mixes. For example, the pancake in the previous menu can contain increased egg and also dried milk to make it contribute at least an additional 4 g of protein in one pancake alone. Instant dried milk has about 1½ g of protein per tablespoonful. At least twice to three times as much dried milk can be used in a flour mixture as is required by the fluid milk equivalent. The use of Canadian bacon or ham instead of bacon would further increase the protein content to approximately one-third of the amount recommended per day for this age child, which is the correct proportion to be served at breakfast.

A word of caution needs to be included to emphasize that fortification of food should be practiced only when needed; food should not be fortified in general without evidence to show that a need exists. Overnutrition should be avoided for intake of protein as well as for other nutrients. Highly questionable dietary practices include such concepts as "if a little bit is good, a lot is better," "better too much than too little," "eat enough for tomorrow too," and others. At times, individuals from war-torn areas suffered deprivation of food to a point that they grossly overate; in their support of gluttony, they declared, "I am not going to die hungry." Such gluttony has no support, neither for protein nor for calories, mineral elements, or vitamins. Neither food fortification nor dietary supplementation should be practiced without careful analysis of dietary intakes. Estimates of dietary intakes based on calculations from food composition tables are reasonably accurate.

Protein requirements are expressed in different ways; the one used by the National Research Council in specifying the Recommended Dietary Allowances (RDA) is "as grams per day for the reference person" at different ages. Such a quantity "as grams per day" does not allow for variations among persons of different size which includes both the concept of total body mass and that of high metabolic tissue or muscularity. Since muscles utilize the major portion of the energy expenditure, protein requirements can be given as grams per kilogram body weight per day or as percentage of energy expenditure (calories metabolized). Some advantages have been found in the use of these two approaches to planning menus or dietary regimen for individuals. A 147-pound man, 18–22 years old has a recommended protein intake of 60 g. If a man of the same age weighed 175 pounds, was nonobese and heavy muscled, his protein as well as calorie needs would be greater and in proportion to the greater muscular mass. Thus dietary recommendations for protein are best specified per unit of size and body composition.

Activities for Student Learning

1. Obtain a standard biochemistry textbook and read about the Kjeldahl method to determine the nitrogen content of a protein or food.
2. Prepare a visual aid demonstrating zero, positive, and negative nitrogen balance.
3. Plan and calculate the protein and calorie content of a one day's menu to meet the protein requirements for a family with four members at different ages or health conditions. Calculate individual amounts of food and compare with the RDA for each person.
4. The following films are recommended for viewing while studying this section on protein:

   "Hungry Angels," No. DK511   "PKU Detection in Oregon"
   from   from
   Association — Sterling Films   Texas State Department of
   8615 Directors Row   of Health
   Dallas, Texas 75247   410 East 5th Street
                                   Austin, Texas

5. Remember to record:

   Hot Tips:

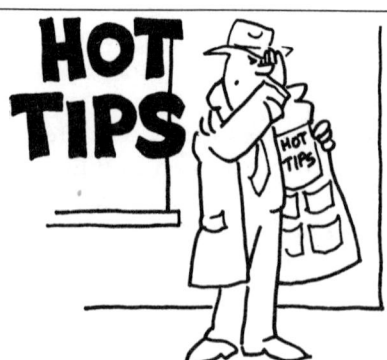

New Words:

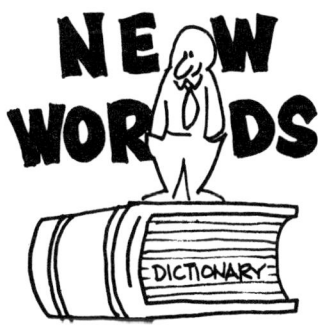

PROTEINS IN FOODS

Objectives

1. To recognize and understand that the amino acid pattern of a food determines the quality of protein in food.
2. To be able to plan and select adequate food sources of dietary protein to meet the daily needs of various individuals of different ages and physiological conditions.
3. To be cognizant of new protein food sources to help meet the world's nutritional needs.

The Amino Acids in Food Proteins

The quantity and quality of the proteins in food determines to some degree the amount of protein needed in the daily diet. A smaller amount of protein of good quality is needed than of protein of poor quality. Quality is determined by the kinds and proportions of the amino acids found in foods.

The quantitative dietary protein requirement of man is still a matter of controversy because of the difficulties involved in experimentation in human nutrition. Far more data are available concerning the requirements for farm and experimental animals than exist for man. The FAO reference pattern was derived from values for the requirements for individual amino acids of mature human subjects and of infants. However, these data represent only a preliminary analysis of the individual needs. Table 7.3 shows the FAO reference protein and the proteins of egg, human milk, and cow's milk compared with the amino acid requirements of infants and adults.

Table 7.3 The FAO pattern and the proteins of egg, human milk, cow's milk, and various legumes as compared with amino acid requirements of human beings.

					Soy				Black[2]	Requirements[1]	
	FAO[1]	Egg[1]	Human[1] milk	Cow's[1] milk	bean[2] meal	Lima[2] beans	Pink[2] beans	Kidney[2] beans	Eyed peas	Infant	Adult
					(g/16 g N) 100 g protein						
Lysine	4.2	6.6	6.6	7.9	6.4	5.9	6.7	7.2	9.6	7.7	5.1
Leucine	4.8	8.8	9.1	10.0	6.6	8.3	9.0	9.1	10.4	10.9	6.6
Isoleucine	4.2	6.6	5.5	6.5	6.4	6.0	6.4	5.5	4.8	6.6	4.6
Methionine	2.2	3.1	2.3	2.5	0.7	1.5	1.2	1.2	0.7	4.8	2.4
Cystine	—	2.3	2.0	0.9	—	—	—	—	—	—	3.5
Total Sulfur a.a.	4.2	5.4	4.3	3.4	—	—	—	—	—	6.2	6.0
Phenylalanine	2.8	5.8	4.4	4.9	4.8	6.2	6.7	6.5	5.7	6.6	2.0
Tyrosine	2.8	5.0	5.5	5.1	3.1	—	—	—	4.7	—	8.0
Total Aromatic	5.6	10.8	9.9	10.0	7.9	—	—	—	—	—	10.1
Threonine	2.8	5.0	4.5	4.7	3.8	4.7	5.2	4.5	3.8	4.4	3.1
Tryptophan	1.4	1.7	1.6	1.4	1.2	0.9	1.2	1.1	1.4	1.6	1.6
Valine	4.2	7.4	6.3	7.0	5.0	7.8	6.4	7.3	5.4	6.7	5.8

[1]Eval. of Pro. Quality., Natl. Acad. Sci., NRC. Pub. 1100, 1963.
[2]Altschul, A. *Processed Plant Protein Foodstuffs*. New York: Academic Press, Inc. 1968, pp. 880–890.

Researchers report determinations of human needs for the essential amino acids. Table 7.4 shows the safe allowances as proposed by Rose (1957) compared to the amino acid content of 100 g edible food portions of some selected foods as reported by Orr and Watt (1957).

Many statements about food composition are misleading unless the food is identified as to ratio of protein, fat and carbohydrate, e.g., whether all edible, raw, or cooked.

Pyke (1970) reported wide variation in the composition of the milk produced by different mammals as can be seen in Table 7.5. The pro-

Table 7.4 Comparison of safe allowances of amino acids with those in selected foods.

Essential amino acids	Safe allowance per day g	Amino acid content of selected foods 100 g edible portion			
		Whole egg	Whole milk	Ground beef	Lima beans
Volume of food		2 med	$\frac{5}{8}$ C	3.8 oz	$\frac{5}{8}$ C
Percentage of protein in food		12.8%	3.5%	16%	20.7%
Lysine	1.6	0.819	0.272	1.398	1.378
Methionine	2.2	0.401	0.086	0.397	0.331
Isoleucine	1.4	0.805	0.223	0.837	1.199
Leucine	2.2	1.126	0.344	1.311	1.722
Phenylalanine	2.2	0.739	0.170	0.658	1.222
Threonine	1.0	0.637	0.161	0.707	0.980
Tryptophan	0.5	0.211	0.049	0.187	0.195
Valine	1.6	0.950	0.240	0.888	1.298
Histidine	—	0.370	0.092	0.556	0.669
Arginine	—	0.840	0.128	1.032	1.315

Table 7.5 Average composition of milk from various animal species (g/100 ml).

	Protein	Fat	Carbohydrate	Calories
Human	1.5	4.0	6.8	68
Elephant	3.5	20.6	7.3	228
Cow	3.5	3.5	5.0	66
Goat	3.7	4.8	4.5	76
Sow	6.2	6.8	4.0	102
Cat	9.0	3.3	4.9	85
Dog	9.9	9.3	3.1	136
Reindeer	10.8	19.6	4.1	234
Rat	11.8	14.8	2.8	192

portion of protein and minerals in the milk of a particular species bears a relationship to the rate of growth of the young of that species.

The protein content of cereal grains varies from 10 to 15%. The amount of protein in the leaves, stems, roots, and fruits of plants is smaller than that found in the various seeds. As shown in Table 7.6, man does not have the capacity to hold sufficient quantity of plant tissue to derive adequate protein intake. Although some of these plants have relatively low yields of protein per serving, their total contribution to meals is considerable for individuals who eat large amounts or eat such foods frequently. Some foods are eaten at every meal and even between meals, whereas others are eaten only at intervals of weeks or months.

Table 7.6   Protein content of various plant tissues.

Part of plant	Example	Protein g/100 g raw EP
Leaves	turnip greens	3.0
	spinach	3.2
Stems	celery	0.9
Tubers	potatoes	2.1
Roots	carrots	1.1
	beets	1.6
Fruits	peaches	0.6
	raisins	2.5
Seeds		
Legumes:		
immature	green peas	3.4
mature	green peas	24.1
	common white	22.3
Nuts:	peanuts	26.3
	almonds	18.6
	pecans	9.2
Cereals:	rice, white	6.7
	rolled oats	14.2
	wheat, rolled	9.9

Meat substitutes and meat extenders.   For the sake of economy and variety in the daily menu, the use of meat substitutes and meat extenders can be employed. In order for a food to be called a meat substitute, it should be similar to meat, supply about 20 g of good quality protein per serving, and should be acceptably pleasing to the consumer. Adequate substitutions for one 3–4 oz serving of meat are:

> 3 oz cheddar cheese
> $\frac{1}{2}$ C cottage cheese
> 6 T peanut butter
> $1\frac{1}{2}$ C cooked beans or peas

Meat extenders are those products which are usually cereal or vegetables as sources of proteins in amounts comparable to the meat replaced. These plant foods are used in various amounts that can be combined with a small amount of meat to make a serving which contains about 20 g of protein in an edible product. These are frequently served as casseroles, loaves, patties, meat balls, and similar items. Examples of extenders commonly used are such items as bread or cracker crumbs, cooked cereal, ready-to-serve cereals, cooked soybean grits, rice, macaroni, noodles, spaghetti, and more recently, new products such as cottonseed flour. The following problem illustrates how such a meat extender would be planned, for example: Mrs. Jones had $\frac{3}{4}$ lb of ground meat to use for serving 6 people for dinner. Could she prepare a main course of rice and ground meat that would meet the 20 g of protein needed for each person? An example is given in Table 7.7 which shows how various ingredients contribute to protein content.

Table 7.7 Calculation of protein in meat extender casserole.

Food item	g protein	
$\frac{3}{4}$ lb ground meat	108.0	
6 t fat	—	
2 C cooked rice	8.4	
1 C white sauce	10.0	
6 olives	0.6	
1 egg	6.1	
1 C breadcrumbs	10.0	
	143.1	g of protein in recipe
	6	servings in recipe
	23	g protein per serving
4 oz serv. beef EP	20	g protein per serving

Production of Protein Foods

"All flesh is grass." Actually meat animals are machines for converting plant nutrients into palatable and nutritious meat, eggs or milk. For example, for each 100 parts of feed energy or calories fed to a pig, 20%

becomes edible pork, a cow will yield 15% as milk, a hen 7% as eggs, a chicken 5% as flesh. In spite of this low conversion ratio of feed to edible animal products, animals will remain as a source of food because of their ability to utilize plant products unacceptable to the digestive mechanism of man. This of course assumes that man would find the plant palatable to his sensory perception. In the category of unacceptable plant tissues are the multiple sources of leaves from grasses, shrubs, legumes, and the like. The highly fibrous celluloses would prove intolerable as would the volume required to furnish the needed total protein. Animals serve a useful function to control much of this leafy vegetation and supply man with variety of food. The United States ranks second to New Zealand in the daily per capita supply of animal protein in comparing the protein food consumption of 43 countries in the world.

Even though legume seeds cannot compete with grasses in their volume contribution to the world's food production, they do have two to four times the protein content of grasses and are critically important in human nutrition when eaten directly as food for man. Grains and legumes are the mainstays of the vegetable portion of man's diet on a global basis, even though a vast variety of other plants are cultivated and consumed.

Lately, a great deal of publicity has been given to the "Green Revolution," an agricultural transformation which is to help increase production of food in proportion to population growth. The main area of hope of this program is in the development and distribution of new high-yield or high-protein strains of food crops. The tale of how the "Green Revolution" happened in the irrigated plains of northern India and in Pakistan was largely responsible for the Nobel Peace Prize being given for the first time to an agriculturist, Dr. Norman E. Borlaug. He has been the wheat specialist of the Rockefeller Foundation since 1944 and currently is director of the wheat program of CIMMYT, an international agency for the improvement of wheat and corn around the world and supported by Rockefeller and Ford Foundations and U.S. State Department's Agency for International Development. Borlaug's work has changed spring wheat yields in India from 10 to 20 bushels per acre to 60 to 70 and even to 100 bushels. Many leaders in analysis of the world economy feel that at best, the "Green Revolution" only buys time for the population growth to be brought under control say by 1980. No increases in food production are sufficient without a corresponding control of population growth in spite of the slogan, "Before peace in the world, there must be food." Even though there seems to be no limit to the advances that are made by agricultural and food technologists, the question remains, how much more improvement in food production can be made? In order to meet the increasing needs of vastly expanding populations and their increasing levels of aspirations, searches for "new proteins" are currently underway in vast numbers of laboratories throughout the United States and the entire world.

Table 7.8 shows that United States households in 1965 spent the highest percentage of their food dollar for all types of meats which supplied the highest percentage of dietary protein and fat. Only the miscellaneous food group approaches the amount of fat supplied by meats but no protein. Grain products and milk products supplied about an equal portion of the family's intake of protein.

As reported by the USDA, "the whole game is replacing expensive meats with inexpensive ones or meat alternatives to supply a like amount of protein" as indicated in Table 7.9.

Table 7.8 Money value and nutrients by food groups.*

Food Group	Percentage of total food				
	Money value	Food energy	Carbohydrate	Fat	Protein
Milk, cream cheese	12.6	12.7	8.7	14.5	20.2
Meats, all sources	32.7	22.3	0.3	37.7	41.6
Other protein foods (includes eggs and legumes)	5.2	5.5	2.7	6.8	10.6
Grain, all products	12.3	25.6	43.4	8.9	19.7
Vegetables and fruits	19.6	9.5	19.0	2.2	6.7
Miscellaneous	17.5	24.4	25.9	30.0	1.4

*USDA. Dietary levels of households in the United States, Spring 1965. U.S. Government Printing Office ARS Report No. 6, 1969.

New Sources of Protein Foods

The *"new protein"* is a product based on an amino acid combination from different proteins, or a combination of different proteins that complement each other nutritionally. In the past, the "nutritional complexity" of natural foods provided an approach to balanced nutrition. With "fabricated or engineered foods," the possibility looms that food processing may jeopardize the nutritional quality of food supply for the consumer by insufficient testing of a new mixture in order to establish its biological value. On the other hand, the mixture may be superior to the natural food and enhance the nutritional supply for the consumer. A great disparity exists in the distribution of proteins around the world

Table 7.9   Comparative costs of 20 grams of protein at June 1970 prices.

Item	Retail price per pound	Cost of 20 g of protein
	Dollars	*Dollars*
Dry beans	0.19	0.04
Peanut butter	0.63	0.10
Chicken, whole, ready-to-cook	0.41	0.12
Eggs, large	0.51 (doz)	0.12
Beef liver	0.68	0.16
Hamburger	0.66	0.17
Tuna fish	0.39 (6½ oz can)	0.17
American processed cheese	0.50 (8 oz pkg)	0.19
Ham, whole	0.78	0.27
Round steak	1.30	0.30
Frankfurters	0.84	0.31
Bologna	0.56 (8 oz)	0.42
Rib roast of beef	1.10	0.42
Bacon, sliced	0.97	0.46

From Food and Home Notes. USDA 3534-70, Washington, D.C.

as well as in the predominant supply of food which serves as the source of protein in each climatic area, e.g., different species of cereals and legumes. But with today's technology, the possibility has developed to fortify cereals and other plant sources of marginal protein quality with lysine and other compounds to make their amino acid profile closely resemble that of dried milk and whole egg. Thus, because the various sources of protein can be made about equal to eggs in nutritional quality, we can speak of "new proteins." An understanding of "new proteins" may bring a clearer understanding between the factors which nourish a consumer and those factors which please his palate and otherwise tempt his impulse to select desirable, convenient, easy-to-prepare, ready-to-eat items.

Many food proteins become candidates for use as "new proteins" depending upon the functional characteristics that are desired for certain food products. Naturally, if these "new proteins" are to be desirable for people, any food products that are developed should furnish both a proper nutritional balance and satisfy a certain place in the dietary habits of the consumers. Some of these that will probably be making headway in the food markets in the near future are:

1. Fish protein concentrate is an inexpensive, stable, tasteless, wholesome product of high nutritive value, prepared from fish under strict controlled sanitary conditions.

2. Oilseed proteins include those from soy, glandless cottonseed, Liquid Cyclone Process (LCP) cottonseed flour concentrate, coconut, sunflower, and rapeseed.
3. Leaf proteins can be extracted from the green leaves of various types of vegetation but are now considered useless or suitable only for feeding to animals.
4. Single-cell organisms such as yeast, bacteria, algae, and fungi are grown on hydrocarbons or carbohydrate waste products from agriculture, lumber, and oil industries.
5. Chemical synthesis of amino acids and polymers of amino acids can be used as supplements to relatively abundant supplies of low quality proteins.

Are there other protein food sources? Western man claims that his food choices are based on rational considerations. Frederick Simoons in his book, *Eat Not This Flesh*, asks the question, "Does it make any better sense to reject nutritious dogflesh, horseflesh, grasshoppers and termites as food than to eat beef or chicken flesh?" It has been pointed out that there are over two million known species of animals; only 50 of these are domesticated and eaten. Of the 250,000 known varieties of vegetables, only 600 are cultivated.

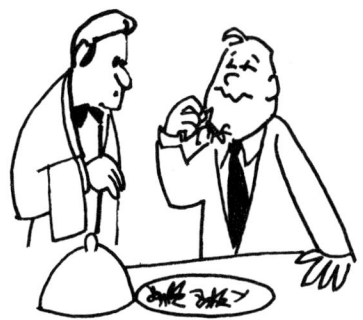

Fig. 7.5 Grasshoppers contain valuable proteins.

Few people realize the extent to which our daily diet is restricted by religious taboos, custom, and tradition. Geography, too, exerts a fundamental influence on food patterns of people restricted to a certain region. Many foods are palatable and nutritious and are significant in the diets of people. The analysis of food habits and food patterns of people in various areas of the world can be fascinating and revealing. The traditional diets differ tremendously, from the East African Masai diet of berries, grain, vegetables, milk and blood from cattle, to the Polynesian diet of coconut, fish, breadfruit, taro, and tropical fruits with pork or poultry occasionally. American and European diets have grown in the past generation to include a fantastic array of foods from all parts of the world. Claims have been made that the striking differences in the state of health and in the physique of people of many nations can be found to correlate with the amount of animal protein consumed in their diets. Such contrasts can be seen by comparing the tall, vigorous, and healthy Pastoral Masai of Kenya who eat large amounts of milk, blood, and flesh to the smaller, weaker, less resistant to tropical diseases Kikuyu tribe of Kenya who eat largely agricultural products of millet, maize, and sweet potatoes. Many other examples can be easily found in studying the cultural, social, and dietary customs of various peoples and locales. The most recent data on the influence of a high cereal diet as compared to one containing more animal protein products were reported on changes in Japanese children by Greulich (1957).

Activities for Student Learning

1. Make a bar graph of the following foods arranged in descending order of protein content: cooked hamburger, cooked pork chop, cooked chicken thigh, baked beans, milk, bread, cottage cheese, apple, potato, and turnip greens.
2. Browse through new journals on food science and technology to keep abreast of new food products that are being developed.
3. Compare the nutritional contribution of animal and plant protein; identify some sources of plant proteins of high biological value.
4. Read biographies of agriculturists who have contributed to increased food production, e.g., Norman Borlaug, E. T. Mertz, N. W. Pirie, Magnus Pyke, and others.

References and Suggested Readings

Altschul, A. *Processed Plant Protein Foodstuffs.* New York: Academic Press, 1968.

Berry, H. K., Hunt, M. M., and Sutherland, B. K. Amino acid balance in the treatment of phenylketonuria, *J. Amer. Dietet. Assoc.,* **58,** 210 (1971).

Chaney, M. S., and Ross, M. L. *Nutrition,* 8th ed. Boston: Houghton-Mifflin, 1971.

Clark, H. E., Mertz, E. T., and Yang, S. P. Influence of caloric intake on urinary nitrogen excretion of men, *Federation Proc.,* **17,** 473 (1958).

Dietary levels of households in the United States, Spring 1965, USDA, ARS. (July 1969).

Fisch, R. O., Solberg, J. A., and Borud, L. Response of children with phenylketonuria to dietary treatment, *J. Amer. Dietet Assoc.,* **58,** 32 (1971).

Greulich, W. W. A comparison of the physical growth and development of American-born and native Japanese children, *Amer. J. Phys. Anthro.,* **15,** 489 (1957).

Harden, M. L., Bush, A., Lamb, M. W., and Yang, S. P. Protein quality of cottonseed flour, *Federation Proc.,* **20:** 2, 297 (1971).

Harden, M. L., and Lamb, M. W. The nutritional value of fractions of the grain sorghum kernel, *Proceedings: 5th World Cereal and Bread Congress,* Dresden, Germany, **6:** 4, 141 (1970).

Harper, A. E. Some implications of amino acid supplementation, *Amer. J. Clin. Nutr.,* **9,** 533 (1961).

Jelliffe, D. B. The assessment of nutritional status, *WHO Chronicle,* **21,** 127 (1967).

Knox, W. E. What's new in PKU, *N. Engl. J. Med.*, **283**, 1404 (1970).

Lowenberg, M. E., Todhunter, E. N., Wilson, E. D., Feeney, M. C., and Savage, J. R. *Food and Man*. New York: Wiley, 1968.

McCance, R. A., and Willowson, E. M., Nutrition and growth, *Proc. Roy. Soc.*, London, **156**, 326 (1962).

Munro, H. N., and Allison, J. B. *Mammalian Protein Metabolism*, Vol. I, II. New York: Academic Press, 1964.

National Academy of Sciences, *Evaluation of Protein Quality*, N.R.C. Pub. 1100, Washington, D.C., 1963.

Orr, M. L., and Watt, B. K. *Amino Acid Content of Food*, Home Eco. Res. Rep. No. 4, USDA, Washington, D.C., 1957.

Passwater, R. A., and Welker, P. A. *American Laboratory*, **5**, 21 (1971).

Pyke, M. *Man and Food*, World University Library. New York: McGraw-Hill, 1970.

Review: Nutrition and mental development, *Dairy Council Digest*, **37**: 5 (1966).

Rose, W. C. Amino acid requirements of adult man, *Nutr. Abstr. & Rev.*, **27**, 631 (1957).

Schaefer, A. E., and Johnson, O. C. Are we well fed? The search for the answer, *Nutr. Today*, **4**: 1, 2 (1969).

Scrimshaw, N. S., and Behar, M. Malnutrition in underdeveloped countries, *N. Engl. J. Med.*, **272**: 137, 193 (1965).

Simoons, F. J. *Eat Not This Flesh*. Madison, Wisc.: Univ. of Wisconsin Press, 1961.

Snider, N. Soy protein: Food service's new staple?, *Inst.* **67**, 125 (1970).

Streeter, C. P. The wheat breeder who won the peace prize, *Farm J.*, 16 (December 1970).

Yang, S. P., Dutton, R. E., Harden, M. L., and Briley, M. E. Effect of amino acid and protein supplementation on the nutritional value of grain sorghum, *Federation Proc.*, **30**: 2, 298 (1971).

INVENTORY OF KNOWLEDGE

Part I

Of the solutions suggested, select the one which best describes present understandings about protein.

1. In world nutrition, protein supply is an acute problem because:
   (a) plants do not normally synthesize protein
   (b) the body's need for protein is more urgent than for other nutrients
   (c) animal sources are unpalatable to most people
   (d) plant life is less efficient than formerly
   (e) animals as suppliers of high quality protein have a low conversion rate of *feed* to food

2. Since proteins are classified on the basis of their chemical and physical makeup, simple proteins are those which:
   (a) contain metallic elements such as iron, copper, etc.
   (b) combine with lipids such as lecithin or cephalin
   (c) yield only amino acids or their derivatives upon hydrolysis
   (d) function in cell nuclei such as DNA
   (e) are formed by hydrolytic cleavage of peptide bonds

3. Protein molecules are characterized by their:
   (a) size comprised of many units of most of the amino acids
   (b) ready solubility in all body fluids
   (c) stable, nonreactive properties
   (d) ease of degradation during digestion
   (e) ready supply of energy for endothermic reactions

4. The efficiency of any "complete protein" can be reduced by:
   (a) subadequate level of protein intake
   (b) eating the wrong accessories with it
   (c) consuming it in excess of needs
   (d) the handling of the food
   (e) dissolving into washing water

5. In order that protein may serve most efficiently for growth, the energy needs of the person should be furnished primarily by:
   (a) carbohydrates and fat
   (b) protein alone
   (c) a larger percentage of calories from protein than from fat
   (d) higher fat than carbohydrate intake
   (e) whatever ratio one prefers

6. A dietary practice to assure adequate amount and quality protein in *low cost menus* is to:
   (a) buy plenty of fresh milk
   (b) choose enough fruit and vegetables
   (c) choose enriched cereals
   (d) use sufficient amounts of vitamins in the diet
   (e) extend inexpensive cuts of meats with cereal products

7. As compared with that of the adult, the protein requirement of the child is:
   (a) the same per kg of body weight
   (b) lower per kg of body weight
   (c) higher per kg of body weight
   (d) not related to age
   (e) dependent on height

Part II

Complete the meaning of the following fragmentary statements by supplying the word, phrase, or term required:

8. The meaning of the term "amino acid supplementation"____

9. An example of the "complementary values of foods as sources of protein"____

10. An early sign of protein deficiency in college-age women____

11. A method used to establish the *biological value* of a protein____

12. The meaning of the term "limiting amino acid"____; the first limiting amino acid in corn and other cereals has been proved to be____

13. The food group to supply the major amount of protein in American dietaries and the amounts of food required____

14. Name and location of a proteolytic enzyme involved in digestion of food____

15. The structure in the cell which degradates large molecules____

16. The first step in metabolism of amino acids occurs

17. The role of DNA and RNA in protein synthesis____

Part III

The following represent numerical relationships; please indicate the procedure used and answer for each situation.

18. Calculate the protein content of the following breakfast and evaluate its adequacy in protein for the normal adult female:

    1 egg (48 g egg; 12% protein)
    2 slices toast (50 g; 8% protein)
    1 glass milk (8 oz or 224 g and average protein)

    What percentage of the RDA for a 55 kg woman is furnished by this breakfast?

8

Mineral Elements in Human Nutrition

Why is the Need to Study Inorganic Nutrients Crucial to People?

An exciting new innovation to the study of minerals is the realization that mineral elements can be either components of rocks and structures of the earth and moon of ash or pumice, or they can be part of the structures of living cells in bone, muscle, and brain. They can be combined with protein, carbohydrates, or lipids to produce needed metabolic catalysts, and they can function as electrolytes in body fluids. Only 4% of the human body weight is composed of mineral elements, which indicates the minute amount of these 14 different inorganic nutrients that have been identified as necessary to function in the body for health and growth.

INORGANIC NUTRIENTS IN THE HUMAN BODY

Objectives

1. To recognize that mineral elements and compounds are essential in different forms to sustain human life.
2. To identify the factors which control the absorption and utilization of mineral elements in the human body.
3. To comprehend the interrelated functions of mineral elements in building body tissues, complex compounds with proteins, lipids and carbohydrates, and in contributing to the composition of body fluids.

Specificity of Function of Mineral Elements

Mineral elements are interrelated to each other and to the organic compounds; the deficiency of one element will affect the functioning of others. The amount of an element present in the body does not designate its importance; a minute quantity of one is as essential as greater quantities of others.

An approach of presenting the interrelated functions of the different mineral elements is presented in Table 8.1. The degree of solubility of the mineral compound relates to its use in the human body. Relatively insoluble compounds such as apatite are necessary for ossification of bones and teeth which form the skeletal structures of the body, while

Table 8.1   Interrelated functions of different mineral elements.

Functions	Mineral Elements*
I. Insoluble compounds as part of the skeleton and other tissues:	
(a) Apatite — insoluble mineral	Calcium-phosphate-fluoride complex deposited in bone and tooth cells; 99% of the body's Ca and 85% of P in this form
(b) Protein in hair, nails, and skin	Sulfur in the amino acids, cystine and methionine, is part of the protein structure
II. Complex organic compounds containing mineral elements:	
(a) Protein-mineral complex in blood, muscles, nerves	Fe in hemoglobin = 60% body's iron
	Fe in myoglobin = 40% body's iron
	P in every cell in complex enzymatic functions as ATP, RNA, etc., in riboflavin
	S as component in amino acids, cystine and methionine; in the vitamin, thiamine; in enzyme systems such as glutathione, in cytochrome, etc.; in the hormone, insulin; in the pigment, melanin
	I in thyroxin
(b) Lipid-mineral complexes	P in lecithins, cephalins
(c) Glyco-mineral complexes	P in phosphogluconate pathway
(d) Other compounds	Co in vitamin B_{12} or cyancobalamin
	Mo in zanthine oxidase
	Se in tocopherol compounds
III. As solutes and electrolytes in solution in body fluids	Previously named elements occur in lesser concentrations, such as Ca^{++}, PO_4^{----}, etc.
	Na^+, and Cl^- ions in interstitial fluids and serum
	K^+ and Cl^- in intracellular fluids

*Symbols are standard for names of chemical elements and are given in Appendix C, pp. 272–273.

some complex organic compounds, solutes and electrolytes, are more reactive and soluble in certain media in order to perform their specific functions.

The absorption of mineral elements differs from that of organic nutrients, varies among the elements, and fluctuates in people. The mineral element has to be released from its structural and chemical involvement in the food and to be made soluble in the gastro-intestinal fluids. Therefore, absorption is relatively inefficient; 20–30% of ingested calcium and 10% of ingested iron are absorbed on average. The balance is nonabsorbed and is excreted in the feces; however, sodium and potassium are usually 100% absorbed. Various factors affect availability and absorption of mineral elements.

Characteristics of food which influence absorption:

1. High cellulose content of diet causes reduced absorption due to hypermotility of gastro-intestinal (G-I) tract, the rate of release of mineral elements from the cellulose complex, and the form in which the element is chemically combined in food.
2. Certain compounds in food, i.e., oxalic acid and phytic acid, form insoluble calcium oxalate and phytate which are excreted in the feces.
3. Certain methods of food preparation reduce the mineral content of edible portions of food.
   Discarding juices and using excessive water in cooking discards up to 50% of mineral content dissolved in juices.
   High temperature with longer than needed time makes protein less digestible with its mineral content nonabsorbable.

Dietary factors which influence absorption:

1. Deficiency of ascorbic acid or of citrus fruits in general decreases absorption.
2. Deficiency of protein for the formation of protein-mineral complexes such as hemoglobin, insulin, thyroxin, etc., results in lowered absorption.
3. Deficiency of lactose or lactic acid reduces absorption of mineral elements.
4. High fat intake may cause formation of insoluble saponified mineral-soap complexes in the G-I tract which prevent absorption.
5. Consumption of dietary mineral supplements with regular meals usually improves absorption but exceptions can occur.

Conditions of G-I tract which influence absorption:

1. Achlorhydria or hypogastric acidity reduces solubility of all mineral elements; this condition can occur when alkaline substances are taken or in older age when hydrochloric acid is reduced.
2. Hypermotility (diarrhea or the effect of laxatives) reduces the time available for absorption and may reduce the efficiency of the intestinal mucosa.

Table 8.2   Schematic diagram of mineral utilization.

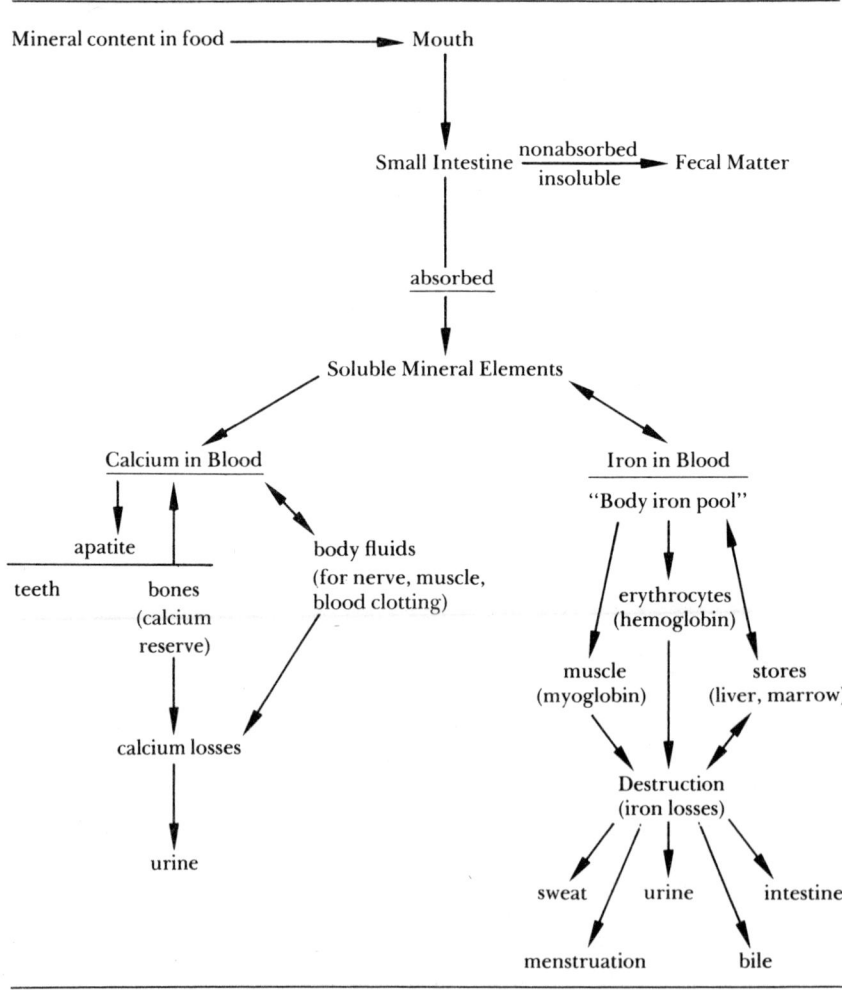

3. Absence of other nutrients essential for absorption, e.g., vitamin D for Ca and P, Cu for iron, etc. can cause reduced absorption.

Body need affects absorption:

1. Pregnancy increases absorption of elements.
2. Following periods of deprivation and starvation, higher absorption occurs.
3. Reduced absorption with increased age is due to multiplicity of factors.
4. Prolonged bed rest or other immobility increases loss of mineral elements from the body which are not replaced by increased absorption.
5. Decreased hormone production with increased age or stress of surgery decreases absorption.

The progressive steps in the utilization of minerals in foods are shown in Table 8.2. During digestion, minerals are separated from the foods eaten and are absorbed through the intestinal wall into the bloodstream to be taken to the areas in the body where they are needed.

DIETARY MINERAL SUPPLY AND THE DEVELOPMENTAL STAGE OF THE INDIVIDUAL

Objectives

1. To compare the mineral element requirements of individual people in the different developmental stages.
2. To recognize the influence of adequate dietary intake of mineral elements upon proper bone and tooth development.
3. To be aware of the influences of dietary intake of people of various ages on blood and body fluid composition.

Influence of Dietary Intake

Many mineral elements are needed for good nutrition; for the normal adult a state of equilibrium, or zero balance where the intake equals the amount excreted, is desirable. During growth, pregnancy, and lactation and other special stress situations, a positive balance of mineral elements is needed to allow the body to build new tissue.

The Food and Nutrition Board of the National Academy of Sciences periodically revises the RDA for various nutrients and age categories to be used as guides in planning and evaluating diets. Currently, the five mineral elements included are calcium, phosphorus, iodine, iron, and magnesium. The elements copper, fluorine, chromium, cobalt, manganese, molybdenum, selenium, and zinc are essential as are the electrolytes sodium, potassium, and chloride but no RDA for them has been established.

The mineral elements most commonly associated with dietary deficiencies in the United States are calcium and iron, and iodine, in some particular geographic areas. Specific planning of menus is necessary to insure the amounts of these minerals needed by the various family members. Major influences of limited intake of these mineral elements can be observed in bone and tooth development and maintenance, dental and oral health, and composition of body fluids.

Bone and Tooth Development and Maintenance

The formation of bone is a highly complicated process, which continues throughout life and occurs predominantly in the epiphyseal area involving the trabeculae of the heads of long bones with the shaft showing less dramatic change. An adequate supply of nutrients is required for normal growth of the skeleton throughout childhood and adolescence. When maturity is reached, no further increase in length of bones occurs although small increases in diameter may occur. Even the adult bone is constantly being resorbed and rebuilt; thus the need for bone building nutrients in the diet continues throughout life.

Bone has the vital functions of providing the rigid framework of the body, serving as a mineral reservoir, and as one of the hematopoietic organs. Bone is a highly specialized form of connective tissue. The hardness results from the deposition of a complex mineral substance within a soft organic matrix of fibrous protein. This deposit is composed chiefly of calcium phosphate, carbonate, and citrate with small amounts of other ions such as sodium, magnesium, and fluoride. In Fig. 8.1 the progression of the growth of bone is illustrated.

Abnormality of bone can develop at any age. In childhood, this manifests itself as sore, tender, and often swollen joints which precede the enlargement at the joints such as the knees, the bending of bones, and malalignment of the skeleton in general. Since the ends of immature bones are the centers of growth and metabolic activity and depend on abundant blood and enzymatic control, these are the focal point of symptoms of dietary deficiency. Naturally, the ends are part of the joints in the skeleton which may carry the whole weight of the body and first show outward signs of dietary deficiency referred to as rickets. The

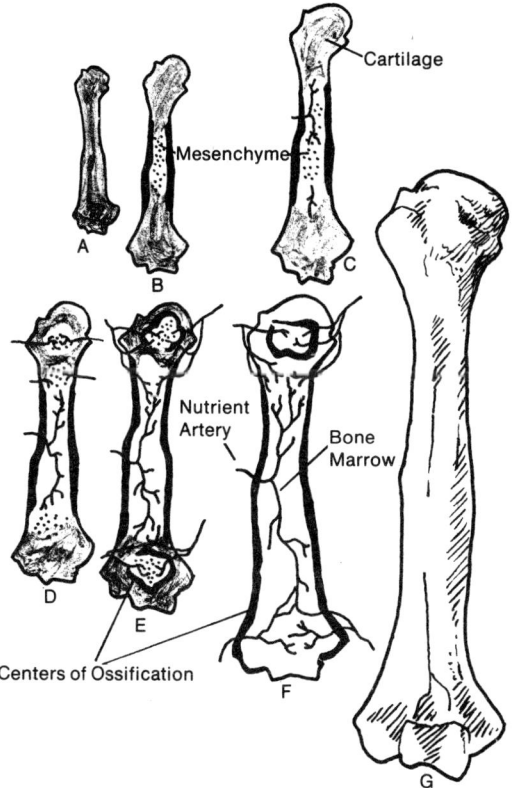

Fig. 8.1   Stages in the development of a typical long bone.
(A)   the original matrix of cartilage
(B)   and (C) a fibrous membrane develops from cartilage and blood vessels and mesen-
chyme invade the structure
(D)   cartilage continues to form at the ends to extend the bone growth gradually to adult
size
(E)   ossification of structure continues at the end or head of the bone and on the outside
of the shaft portion
(F)   the circulatory system carries dissolved materials from the interior bone marrow
region to the exterior of the bone, allowing the interior space to increase in size in
proportion to the exterior, i.e., the hollow area increases in ratio to the size of the
bone
(G)   the mature bone

so-called "growing pains" of childhood could easily be related to these
bone anomalies commonly referred to as subclinical rickets, resulting in
reversible or even irreversible bone deformity.

In adults with rigid bones and a minimum of cartilage, bone abnormalities can exist unnoticed for years and may be associated with pains in the joints or in muscles and collectively referred to as rheumatism or arthritis. Careful medical examinations with analyses of blood and urine can identify osteomalacia and osteoporosis. These conditions may have progressed during years of marginal dietary intakes of several nutrients including calcium, phosphorus, vitamins A, D, and C, and even protein. Changes in posture, gait, and feeling of well-being progress gradually until disaster occurs resulting in a bone fracture which can neither be "pinned" nor will heal effectively. The concept currently held is that all too often a fracture occurs and the individual falls rather than vice versa. Undoubtedly, the hunched back of aging people is related to spongy, collapsing vertebrae as well as to weakened muscularity to hold the body erect. Residents in nursing and convalescent homes attest to the frequency of this disaster occurring mostly to women after menopause. Rather indefinite results are obtained with sex hormone therapy, even though undoubtedly this is involved in addition to dietary inadequacies.

Dental decay is probably the most prevalent disease affecting all mankind. In the United States, 98% of the population has dental caries during the life-span. Most people are unaware that all dental decay and most peridontal disease are preventable. The effects of nutrition on oral health can best be observed in these two areas: *dental caries* more prevalent in youth and *peridontal disease* in later years.

Structurally sound teeth are formed prior to the mid-teen years if optimum nutrition and other conditions were prevalent during this early period of development. Several nutrients are involved in tooth development:

> *protein* for the matrix formation;
>
> *calcium, phosphorus,* and *vitamin D* (under influence of parathyroid glands) for deposition of the mineral compound, apatite, into the matrix structure;
>
> *ascorbic acid,* involved in mineral element utilization and for cementum formation to connect the tooth to the bone structure and to the gum tissues;
>
> *vitamin A* concerned with proper functioning of enamel-forming cells to achieve a smooth, even enamel layer as well as a deposit of sound dentine; and
>
> *fluorine* contributes to hardening the enamel making it resistant to cariogenesis.

Since permanent teeth erupt full adult size, they may seem disproportionately large for the jaw and face and may appear to crowd the teeth to cause malalignment or malocclusion for a short time. The face soon grows to match the teeth, which if properly formed and cared for should remain in the jaw for the duration of life. The six-year molars are the most neglected permanent teeth, since many parents do not realize that they are not temporary teeth.

Oral health involves the control of the environment of the teeth so that they can survive the longest period of any body tissue. All body tissues undergo dynamic exchange of molecules; e.g., the erythrocytes are completely replaced every six weeks. Teeth, because of their density and chemical structure, have a very slow rate of exchange and therefore survive for the longest period of time. No evidence exists to indicate that a tooth can repair itself, or that decay occurs from within; tooth decay occurs exclusively on the surface of the tooth — due to some corrosive action. This action may be either mechanical, such as repeated scrubbing with abrasive substances harder than the tooth like powdered pumice, or chemical which is mostly the action of an acid or enzyme on a mineral salt. The origin of the irritant may be either food, drink, or may be from the metabolism of bacteria living on food residues (especially sugar) left between teeth, in crevices, or at the gumline. These are all involved in dental plaque formation and caries production.

The development of dental caries is recognized as an infection caused by a group of bacteria; it is a disease. The dentist has the responsibility to prevent this disease in addition to repair of caries already in progress. Tooth decay entails a combination of three processes simultaneously:

1. demineralization of the inorganic enamel structure,
2. proteolytic breakdown of the organic matrix of the dentine, and
3. an invasion by the cariogenic bacteria of the dentinal tubules.

The cariogenic organism acts specifically on carbohydrate, especially on sucrose, which gives sugar the highest cariogenicity of any dietary substance. Stahl (1969) summarizes that nutritional deficiencies do not initiate peridontal disease but do contribute delay in healing and repair of gingival tissue. The type of diet eaten and the overall dietary practices affect oral health not only through physiological processes, but also by external influences on teeth and gums.

Recently, interest has centered on dental plaque formation which is considered to be related to both tooth decay and peridontal disease. Research supports the hypothesis that sucrose, especially in adhesive sticky foods, supports bacterial growth with subsequent plaque formation, caries development, and eventually peridontal problems. The frequency of eating sweets appears to be the focal point and not the amount eaten. Thus dental decay is an environmental problem of teeth in which dental plaque formation is produced by sucrose and bacteria and reduced by an environment containing calcium and phosphate ions.

Progression of tooth decay occurs in those areas in which sugar residues collect and plaque formation escapes oral hygiene tactics. As Fig. 8.2 illustrates, the vulnerable areas are the surface crevices of molars and the gumline deposits along all teeth but especially for those which are most difficult to cleanse. Also spaces between crooked malaligned teeth have more frequent caries development than properly spaced teeth.

STRUCTURAL PARTS

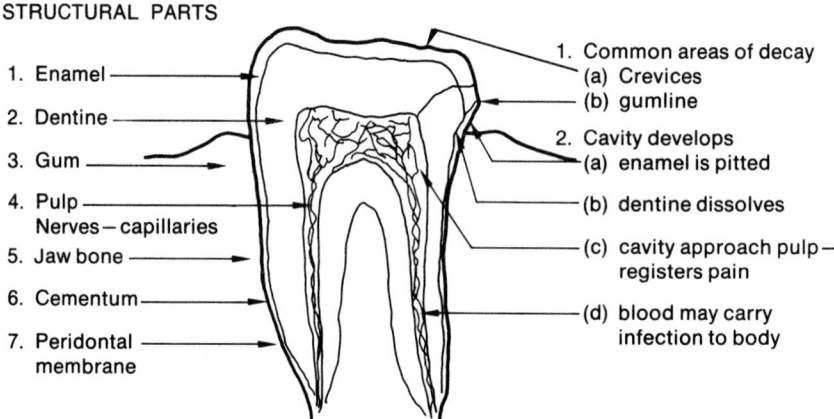

1. Enamel
2. Dentine
3. Gum
4. Pulp
   Nerves – capillaries
5. Jaw bone
6. Cementum
7. Peridontal
   membrane

1. Common areas of decay
   (a) Crevices
   (b) gumline
2. Cavity develops
   (a) enamel is pitted
   (b) dentine dissolves
   (c) cavity approach pulp –
       registers pain
   (d) blood may carry
       infection to body

Fig. 8.2   Tooth decay is related to tooth structure as well as food residues.

The thrust for improvement of dental health should include:

1. Proper dietary practices to avoid adhesive sugar clinging undisturbed to tooth structures for extended periods of time and to supply required nutrients and fibrous foods for oral hygiene.
2. Regular oral hygiene involving prompt cleansing of teeth after eating, considering proper equipment and dentifrices.
3. An organized fluoride supply at one of several points:
   (a) natural concentration of fluorides in a water supply or fluoridated communal water system with a concentration of about one part per million of fluoride,

(b) use of fluoridated dentifrices preferably using stannous fluoride as the additive,
(c) topical application of fluorides directly to the tooth enamel increases its resistance to decay.

Fluoride and Bone and Tooth Maintenance

Fluorine has long been recognized as a normal constituent of bones and teeth, the dental enamel has been found to be especially rich in this nutrient. The enamel surface is capable of taking up fluorine shortly after eruption, the earlier a child has an available source of fluorine, the fewer caries he will develop.

In February 1971, more than 5000 communities in the United States were adding fluorides to their public water supplies at the ratio of one part of fluoride per million parts of water (1 ppm). Each year 400–500 communities initiate the addition to reduce the frequency of dental decay among their populations. In addition, 2624 communities have water supplies with natural fluorine content in subsoil waters. Thus some 88.5 million people in the United States have access to fluoride to increase the resistance of tooth enamel to corrosive action. Repeated surveys have shown that the DMF rate (number of decayed, missing, and filled teeth) prior to and 10 years following fluoridation shows over 60% reduction following fluoridation. For example, a youth with no fluoride in his communal water supply may have 10 cavities, whereas one who had fluoride will have only four. Fluoridated dentifrices reduce decay by 20%.

Naturally, neither fluorides nor any nutrient alone can solve the physiological need of any tissue; the role of each element depends on the adequacy of the diet. Some elements show close association in their function, e.g., phosphates and fluorides work together synergistically to control caries in different ways. The chemical physiology of the surface of the teeth is still a mystery but is being actively investigated.

Furthermore, fluoride has been shown to increase the stability of bones against calcium losses that may occur after menopause, during bedridden confinement, and during immobility such as during space flights. This bone demineralization is less in people with drinking water containing the therapeutic level of fluoride.

Dietary Intake as Related to Blood and Fluid Composition

A major step to improve the nutritional status of American people was made in 1941 with the passage of the War Food Order No. 1, requiring the enrichment of white flour and bread with iron and three vitamins. Undoubtedly this increases the iron intake of people who eat these foods. Nonetheless research continues to show physiological deficits of iron-containing compounds such as hemoglobin in the erythrocytes of the blood of infants, children, and young women. The following are proposed as reasons for the continued nutritional deficit of iron compounds:

1. Very low rates of absorption of iron from dietary food supplies, averaging only about 10% in healthy people; absorption from dietary supplements and pharmaceutical sources may be lower.
2. Continued decreased consumption of foods normally supplying appreciable amounts, namely,
   (a) cereal products, especially whole kernel and enriched ones
   (b) prepared food in which mature, outer leaves richer in iron than immature ones are removed; foods pared to uniform size discarding the mineral-rich layer immediately under the peeling,
   (c) reduced use of utensils and equipment made of iron, which in contact with food possibly allowed some iron to dissolve into the food,
   (d) less soup and stew-type foods featured in menus which often have higher mineral content since the juice is eaten.
3. Increased consumption of "pure food" items as the primary source of calories.
4. Use of limited supply of iron-rich foods, some are avoided such as egg yolks because of cholesterol (atherosclerosis), all meats because of price, small servings in prepared foods, dried beans and mature peas because of purine (gout), others because of cost, fear of calorie content, or family custom.

Further research on enrichment of food must take into consideration the foods which are eaten by those who need the iron. Currently, less than 1% of men have any indication of needing additional iron in their bodies. Children and women need to eat the foods fortified with iron if this technic of dietary improvement is to be effective.

The blood carries nutrients to the various tissues and reflects the dietary supply of many nutrients, some more accurately than others. If a person wants to know himself, he at least should be aware of the normal composition of blood. Table 8.3 is a compilation of the major constituents commonly found in blood "at the fasting level" which is usually after 12–14 hours of no food intake. Absorption of nutrients from a recent meal would quickly alter levels of many nutrients.

Table 8.3   Nutrient constituents of normal blood.

I. Gross Composition of blood:

Cell volume	39–50%
Erythrocytes	4.5–5 million per ml of blood
Hemoglobin (in erythrocytes)	13–17.25 g per 100 ml
Leucocytes	5000–9000 per ml of blood
Platelets	tiny, oval or round disks; thrombocytes
Plasma	fluid portion of blood
Serum	plasma after coagulation of fibrinogen

II. Organic components:

Glucose   *70–90 mg per 100 ml

Lipids   *570–820 mg per 100 ml plasma; neutral fat 154; total fatty acids 353; cholesterol 100–230 mg; phospholipids 196

Amino Acids — (*J. Biol. Chem.*, **188**, 833, 1951.)

mcg per ml of plasma

Arginine	*16.2	Methionine	*5.2
Cystine	*14.7	Phenylalanine	*9.9
Histidine	*13.8	Threonine	*16.7
Isoleucine	*13.4	Tryptophan	*12.7
Leucine	*18.6	Tyrosine	*10.4
Lycine	*21.9	Valine	*27.2

Serum Protein Content

Total	6.5–7.5 g per 100 ml serum
Albumen	4.5–5.5 g per 100 ml serum
Globulin	1.5–2.5 g per 100 ml serum

III. Mineral Elements:

Calcium	9–11 mg per 100 ml blood, 60% of which is in a soluble, ionized form, the balance is bound in protein molecule
Iron	50 mcg per 100 ml plasma (50–180 mcg %); all in the form of hemoglobin
Phosphorus	3–4 mg per 100 ml serum

IV. Vitamins:

Carotene	75–125 mcg per 100 ml
Thiamine	4.7 ± 0.19 mg per 100 ml
Riboflavin	20 mg per 100 ml
Niacin	13 mg per ml
Ascorbic Acid	Saturated 0.75–1.5 mg per 100 ml

Sodium in today's foods. Change in food customs is having detrimental effects on dietary supplies of iron and other nutrients. However, some nutrients may be increased beyond safe limits, namely sodium. At one time sodium was supplied predominantly by table salt (NaCl), with baking soda or baking powder a secondary source. Increased sodium intake is cause for concern since it relates to edema or excessive fluid retention in tissues and to hypertension or high blood pressure. A decade ago diets were specified as "low salt" or "salt free" for certain physiological symptoms; soon the substance involved was identified as sodium rather than salt. Dietitians are amazed to note the supply of this element in diets from sources previously not considered as significant.

One such source is drinking water. Most waters flowing through water softeners of the ionic displacement or zeolite type operate on the basis that the sodium ion replaces the hard water's calcium or magnesium ions. Furthermore, most naturally "soft water" already contains sodium. Sodium is extracted from soil by surface runoff waters, collected in lakes, and used as municipal water.

Food technology uses sodium salts of various compounds as additives which include sodium derivatives such as:

sodiumcyclamate	monosodiumphosphate
sodiumsaccharin	sodium glutamate
sodiumproteinate	sodiumsorbate

These compounds are included in food for a variety of functions which include:

noncalorie sweeteners	flavor enhancers
mold inhibitors	preservatives and
emulsifiers	tenderizers

Dietetic and prepared foods often contain many of these additives and supply sodium in unspecified quantities.

Activities for Student Learning

1. You will need to review and study the physiology of bone formation in a standard textbook on physiology and correlate development to dietary needs.
2. Give examples of the ways in which mineral elements function together in the skeletal structures and in regulatory processes of the body.
3. Please prepare an educational display showing the interrelationships of certain minerals.
4. Could you construct a bingo game or simple crossword puzzle using functions or signs of deficiencies with the mineral elements involved? These could be devices to teach certain nonacademic minded young adults.

References and Suggested Readings

Bronner, F. Fluoridation-Issue on Obsession? *Amer. J. Clin. Nutr.*, **22**: 1346 (1969).

Bullamore, J. R., Gallagher, J. C., Wilkinson, R., Noedin, B. E., and Marshall, D. H. *Lancet 7671*, 535, September 1970.

Caddell, J. L. Magnesium deficiency . . . in extremis, *Nutr. Today*, **2**: 1, 14 (1967).

Division of Dental Health, Public Health Service, *Fluoridation Census, 1969*. U.S. H.E.W., Washington, D.C. (1970).

Finch, C. A. Iron metabolism, *Nutr. Today*, **4**: 2, 2 (1969).

Hartles, K. L. Dietary modification as a means of control of dental caries, *Roy. Soc. of Health J.*, **90**, 316 (1970).

Hegsted, D. M. The recommended dietary allowances for iron, *Amer. J. of Public Health*, **60**, 653 (1970).

Iodized salt, *Nutr. Today*, **4**: 1, 22 (1969).

Krehl, W. A. Magnesium, *Nutr. Today*, **2**: 3, 16 (1967).

Lamb, M. W., and Ford, E. Dental health of children in the fourth grade of four elementary schools in Lubbock, Texas, *J. of School Health*, **30**, 15 (1960).

Martin, P. C., and Vincent, E. L. *Human Development*. New York: Ronald Press, 1960.

Massler, M., Nutrition and dental decay, *Food and Nutr. News*, **39**, 5, National Livestock and Meat Board, Chicago, 1968.

Monsen, E. R. The need for iron fortification, *J. Nutr. Educ.*, **2**: 4, 152 (1971).

Nizel, A. E. Food habits and their modification for caries control, *Nutr. News*, **32**, 1 (1969).

Present Knowledge in Nutrition, 3rd ed. New York: The Nutrition Foundation, 1967.

Review of studies of vitamin and mineral nutrition in the United States (1950–1968), *J. Nutr. Educ.*, **1**, 2, Suppl. 1 (1969).

Robinson, J. Water, the indispensable nutrient, *Nutr. Today*, **5**: 1, 16 (1970).

Sandstead, H. H. Zinc—a metal to grow on, *Nutr. Today*, **3**: 1, 12 (1968).

Sognnaes, R. F. Fluoride protection of bones and teeth, *Science*, **150**, 989 (1965).

Stahl, S. S. Nutritional influences on peridontal disease, *Food and Nutr. News*, **40**, 1 (1969).

Swanson, P. P. *Calcium in Nutrition*, pamphlet. Chicago: National Dairy Council, 1967.

Underwood, E. J. *Trace Elements in Human and Animal Nutrition*. New York: Academic Press, 1962.

Your teeth: Folklore and fallacies, *Today's Health*, 8 (April 1964).

INVENTORY OF KNOWLEDGE

Part I

Choose one of the mineral elements listed on the right for each statement and record its letter in the space provided.

_____ 1. Deficiency results from an exclusive milk diet

_____ 2. Excessive perspiration may cause deficiency

_____ 3. Depletion is readily achieved by hemorrhages

_____ 4. Reduction of intake is recommended in treatment of edema

(a) Calcium (e) Sodium
(b) Iron (f) Fluorine
(c) Phosphorus (g) Other
(d) Iodine

_____ 5. The average absorption rate is about 10%

_____ 6. Hypogastric acidity contributes to low erythocyte levels

_____ 7. Oranges, which enhance absorption, are a unique source

_____ 8. A daily intake of 800 mg is recommended for adults

_____ 9. The compound apatite contains in addition to calcium

_____10. The NRC's RDA for women is much greater than that for men

_____11. An average of 1 mg–1.5 mg is lost during menstruation

_____12. Chronic infection accompanied by achlorhydria increases deficiency

_____13. Recommended intake varies from 10 to 18 mg

_____14. Seafood may be a major dietary supply

_____15. Milk and cheese are most concentrated source

_____16. Hypothyroidism results from deficiency

_____17. Added to "enriched flour and bread"

_____18. A major factor in control of tooth decay

_____19. Spinach, rhubarb, and chocolate contain a substance to decrease solubility

_____20. Dried fruits, especially apricots are a good diet supplement

_____21. Mostly supplied in the consumable water supply

_____22. Adequate intake crucial to dental development prior to adolescence

_____23. Diarrhea and vomiting in infants can cause serious depletion

_____24. Mineral content apt to be low in infant's diet

_____25. Major concentration in human body is an insoluble deposit

Part II

Select the appropriate response:

26. Minerals in solution in body fluids involved in maintaining the osmotic pressure of the membranes are:
    (a) potassium, sodium
    (b) calcium, iron
    (c) sodium, sulfur
    (d) iodine, potassium
    (e) calcium, fluorine

27. The primary reason for fluoridation of communal water is to:
    (a) reduce the susceptibility of the teeth to decay
    (b) reduce the mottling of teeth
    (c) prevent staining
    (d) increase the rate of ossification
    (e) alter structure of the teeth and bones

28. The most significant sources of sodium in the diet are:
    (a) refined products
    (b) fruits and vegetables
    (c) carbonated drinks
    (d) candies
    (e) additives to processed foods

29. The increase in dental caries in underdeveloped countries and the United States is proportional to:
    (a) total calorie intake
    (b) the lack of adequate mineral intake
    (c) scarcity of animal protein
    (d) Vitamin D deficiency
    (e) amount and frequency of consuming refined sugars

30. Suggestions made by dentists to reduce tooth decay are:
    (a) reduce the amount of sweets consumed
    (b) choose more crisp fruits and vegetables
    (c) brush or rinse teeth after eating
    (d) use a fluorinated dentrifice
    (e) all of these

31. The percentage of the RDA for Ca for the average woman, 18–75 years furnished by 3 oz canned salmon with 167 mg Ca:
    (a) 21
    (b) 10
    (c) 15
    (d) 42
    (e) 56

32. The level of fluoride which is recommended to be added to communal water supplies is:
    (a) 10%
    (b) 10 ppm
    (c) 1 ppm
    (d) 0.9%
    (e) 8 ppm.

Part III

The following statements are either true or false; please identify your view with a + for the one you judge to be true and identify what makes the others false.

33. Mineral elements require special digestive enzymes for absorption.

34. Mineral elements such as calcium or iron salts are more soluble in acid solution than in alkaline ones.

35. Generally the functions of minerals are independent of those of other nutrients.

36. Unabsorbed dietary mineral salts are excreted in the feces.

37. The RDA for iron is most readily supplied in women's diets.

38. Adequate amounts of sodium are difficult to supply in modern technology.

39. Mineral elements share a function of maintenance of osmotic pressure.

40. Adequate supplies of potassium accompany adequate intake of plant foods.

41. Sulfur is the most abundant mineral element in the human body.

42. A common insoluble compound in the body is apatite in osteoblastic cells.

43. Cereal products serve as a significant supply of iron in family diets.

44. Thyroxine contains chlorine in its molecular structure.

45. Mothers can increase iron intake of children by using brown sugar and molasses in cookery.

9

Vitamins in Human Nutrition

What Are Vitamins?

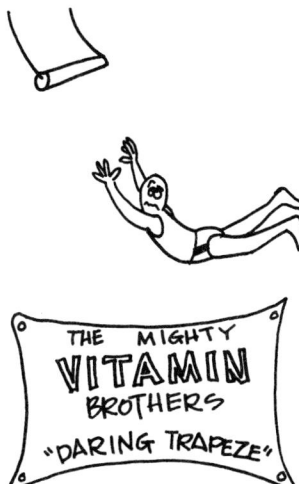

Fig. 9.1 All metabolic processes depend directly or indirectly on vitamins.

The small amount of vitamins that are needed for life gives no clue to their significance; all metabolic processes which develop and maintain every cell in the human body depend on vitamins. Because minute amounts were so easily overlooked, the presence and importance of vitamins were not identified until the early 1900s. Since that time, so much has been written that now names of vitamins are common household words. Vitamins became known by their absence — they were discovered because they were not there — rather like the saying that, "you don't miss the water until the well runs dry."

Vitamins were first called "accessory factors" by Sir Frederick G. Hopkins, British biochemist, who demonstrated in 1906 that normal foods contained minute traces of substances essential to health. The curative effect of certain foods in conditions such as scurvy, rickets, beriberi, pellagra, and various other symptoms observed throughout history were related to these unknown "accessory factors."

CONCEPT OF MICRONUTRIENTS

Objectives

1. To recognize the role of minute quantities of vitamins in human nutrition.
2. To identify man's dependence on other organisms for his survival.

The Significance of Minute Amounts

The vitamin theory of etiology of diseases was revolutionary and even when the vitamins were recognized as being of value in treatment of disease, few observers realized that they were also needed by the normal person. Even for minute amounts of molecules classed together as vitamins, a deficiency of the minute amount would ultimately interfere with the functioning of all other nutrients, since all nutrients participate in the growth and maintenance of the organism.

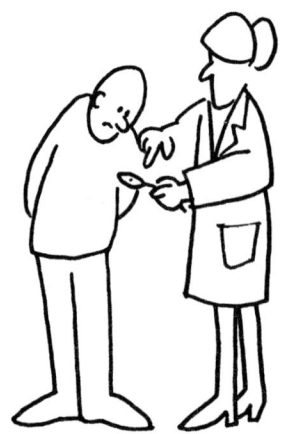

Fig. 9.2 Only a minute amount of any vitamin is required.

People are familiar with quantities of food eaten at a meal and with the smaller amounts eaten by infants and young children. To realize that most of the volume of food eaten is indigestible, namely water, air, cellulose and other indigestible material is surprising but understandable. Again the fact that the nutrients constitute only 12% of milk, 7% of cabbage, or 50% of meat is not generally known. A level teaspoonful of pure carbohydrate, fat or protein which weighs about 4–5 g can be visualized. Can a person really see one thousandth of a fourth of a teaspoon as the amount of thiamine needed for the metabolic production of energy expenditure of 2000 calories? This is the average daily energy expenditure of a young woman weighing 115 pounds and moderately active; to metabolize this amount of energy expenditure, she should consume 1 mg of thiamine. The amount can easily be lost in a crack of the cutting board or spilled into the sink.

The concept of micronutrients opened a whole new set of measurements in human nutrition. Even though many mineral elements are

Table 9.1 Vitamin nomenclature.

Common Name	Date Isolation from Food	Date Chemical Synthesis	Other Names
Fat Soluble Vitamins			
Retinol (Vitamin A)	1932	1947	Antixerophthalmic factor, also axerophythol, retinol, dehydro-retinol, retinoic acid, retinal, dehydroretinal. Vitamin A group includes A_1, A_2, A_{acid}, retinene, and retinene$_2$
Vitamin D	1927	1931	Antirachitic vitamin, also calciferol, viosterol, irradiated ergosterol, ergosterol, ergo-calciferol, cholecalciferol. Vitamin D group includes D_2, D_3, etc.
Vitamin E	1936	1938	Antisterility factor, the tocopherols. Vitamin E group includes alpha, beta, and gamma tocopherols
Vitamin K	1936	1939	Blood clotting factor, koagulations vitamin, anti-hemorrhagic factor, phylloquinone, farnoquinone. Vitamin K group includes K_1, K_2, menadione, etc.
Water Soluble Vitamins			
Ascorbic Acid (Vitamin C)	1918	1933	Antiscorbutic factor, cevitamic acid, Ascorbic acid, vitamin J (vitamin C_2)
B *Complex Group*: B_1 through B_{15}, B_c, B_p, B_t, B_w, B_x, *pantothenic, biotin, choline, inositol, para aminobenzoic acid, and the folic acid group*			
Thiamine	1926	1936	Vitamin B_1, antiberiberi factor or antineuritic factor, aneurine, vitamin F
Riboflavin	1933	1935	Vitamin B_2, vitamin G, lactoflavin, ovoflavin, hepatoflavin, yellow enzyme
Niacin	1913	1938	PP factor (pellagra-preventing), nicotinic acid, anti-black-tongue factor, niacinamide or nicotinamine, vitamin B_3, chick pellagra factor
Pyridoxine	1932 & 1938	1939	Pyridoxol, pyridoxine, vitamin B_6 group (pyridoxal, pyridoxamine, etc.) rat acrodynia factor, adermin, vitamin Y

Table 9.1   *Continued*

Common Name	Date Isolation from Food	Date Chemical Synthesis	Other Names
Cobalamin	1948	1955–56	Antipernicious anemia principle (B_{12a}, B_{12b}, and B_{12d}), cobalamin, cyancobalamin (B_{12}), hydroxo-cobalamin (B_{12b}) nitrocobalamin (B_{12c}), Castles extrinsic factor, the erythrocyte maturation factor, and the animal protein factor (B_{12})
Panthothenic Acid	1933	1940	Pantothen, filtrate factor, chick antidermatitis factor, anti-chromotrichia factor (anti-gray hair factor), vitamin B_x
Biotin	1936	1943	Anti-egg-white injury factor, vitamin H, coenzyme R, bios II, factor S, factor W, factor X, biotinic acid
Choline	1962		Bilineurine
Inositol	1928		Inosite, bios I, mouse antialopecia factor, muscle sugar
Para aminobenzoic acid	1940		PABA
Folacin	1945	1945–48	Pteroylglutamic acid (PGA) folacin; a group known as vitamin R, M, B_c, factor U, *Lactobacillus casei* factor, eluate factor, factor R, vitamin B_{10} and B_{11}, folic acid, folinic acid, citrovorum factor, vitaminM
Vitamin P Group			Bioflavonoids, citrin permeability factors, rutin (no longer considered a vitamin)

only needed in quantities of milligrams, usually these were considered as a composite in ash which could be seen, handled, and understood. When handling vitamins in pharmaceutic preparations, quantities of "filler" are added, not only to help preserve the reactive vitamin in a chemi-cally inert environment of starch, sugar, or other material but also to give the pill, tablet, or capsule enough volume for convenient handling. A person giving an infant his daily dose of vitamins would need to place only a small droplet on the infant's tongue to furnish the daily dietary need in generous amounts. To control the amount given and to help prevent excessive intakes, a diluent is added. Even then the overzealous uninformed person may supply excessive quantities to the helpless child. Such practices are considered the chief cause of hypervitaminosis D, for example.

The micronutrients are as specific in function and as indispensable to the physiological processes of a person as any other essential dietary component. However, they offer a problem of special concern in their retention during the processing and preparation of food for consumption. Some micronutrients are soluble in water and may easily be discarded. In addition to this problem, some readily undergo chemical decomposition when in contact with air, high temperatures, and other environmental conditions.

Alphabetical designations were assigned the micronutrients by early researchers. Considerable concern was expressed in the early 1920s about the name, "vitamine" which the biochemist, Casimer Funk coined in 1911 to mean an amine vital to life. As the chemical nature was identified, various names were designed to identify elements and radical groups within the vitamin molecule as can be seen in Table 9.1.

CHARACTERISTICS OF VITAMINS

Objectives

1. To be aware that chemical properties of the vitamins determine their functions, the food which supplies them, and their retention in food preparation.
2. To comprehend that since vitamins are a chemically heterogeneous group, each has specific physiological functions in that particular organism as all species of animals do not have the same dietary needs.
3. To recognize the functions of vitamins to be comparable to those achieved by metabolic enzymes and hormones, namely, catalysts for specific chemical changes essential for life.

Resemblance of Vitamins to Enzymes and Hormones

These substances have certain characteristics in common:

1. Enzymes, hormones and vitamins are organic compounds synthesized in living plants, are reactive, and deteriorate readily. Vitamins are not synthesized by people and must be eaten regularly.
2. They function in minute amounts measured in milligram and microgram quantities.
3. They are specific in their catalytic action, each has a function or reaction to catalyze which is not possible for another to do.

4. Each requires specific environmental conditions for it to be chemically and physiologically active which controls the locality and the duration it performs.

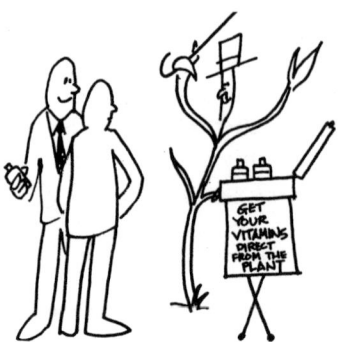

Fig. 9.3 All vitamins are originally synthesized by plants or single cell organisms.

5. Many of the enzymes and hormones have components which must be furnished by the diet, e.g., specific essential amino acids and mineral elements. The basic vitamin must be ingested for it to combine with biological components to perform in the active enzyme systems.

6. All vitamins are originally synthesized by plants or single cell organisms; animals are dependent on plants to furnish these molecules called vitamins.

7. They are deactivated by change in temperature, acidity or alkalinity, and other environmental changes.

Physiological Characteristics of Vitamins

To clarify the characteristics of some 15 vitamins, they are divided into those which are soluble in water and those that are soluble in fats and fat solvents. Since the circulatory medium of the human body is a water solution, the water soluble vitamins, after their release during digestion, are rapidly absorbed by the blood and as rapidly filtered from the blood by the kidneys. The fat soluble group is digested and absorbed via the pathways common to fats or triglycerides. The fat soluble vitamins are stored in the liver and other organs where toxic levels may accumulate. Table 9.2 gives the characteristics of the water and fat soluble vitamins, and Table 9.3 lists some of their specific and related functions.

Clinical Assessment of Vitamin Nutrition

In recent years, researchers have developed technics for determining vitamins in blood cells, plasma and in urine to aid in assessment of the nutritional status of people. Saturation tests can be performed with water soluble vitamins to establish the maximum levels which the blood tolerates and the rate of filtration by the kidneys for excretion of

Table 9.2 Characteristics of the vitamins.

Characteristic	Water Soluble Vitamins	Fat Soluble Vitamins
Symbols	B vitamins, C	A, D, E, K
Chemical elements	Carbon, hydrogen, oxygen; all the B's have nitrogen, B_1 has sulfur, B_{12} has cobalt	Carbon, hydrogen, and oxygen
Sources	All living tissues, involved in energy and in other chemistry of cell life	Not found in all living tissue, but in certain specialized ones such as egg yolk, liver, kidney, fat of milk; concentration is very low in adipose tissue. The precursor of vitamin A is synthesized by plants as certain yellow pigments
Digestion and absorption	Dissolved from food and absorbed through mucosa of the small intestines into the capillaries of the blood	Dissolved in substances that dissolve fat; first these vitamins must be emulsified with fat and have a water soluble carrier; then they are absorbed from the small intestine with fat molecules by the lacteals of the lymph system
Physiological use	B vitamins are interrelated and involved with energy metabolism. Ascorbic acid is involved with polymucosaccharides of cellular metabolism for the production of collagen, an intercellular connective protein	Vitamin A related to the functioning of all epithelial tissues, D is required for absorption and deposition of calcium and phosphorus, E is an antioxidant, and K is involved in prothrombin formation for blood clotting. Amounts required are based on body size
Storage	None; tissues become saturated, any excess is quickly filtered from the blood by the kidneys	In liver, kidney, and other tissues which can result in hypervitaminosis
Toxicity	None reported	Excessive storage has been reported to damage the liver, kidney, and other organs and tissues
Influence of stress such as growth, disease, pregnancy	Increases need	Increases need
Excretion	In urine	In feces

Table 9.3   Functions of selected vitamins.

Vitamins of Dietary Significance	Specific and Related Functions
Vitamin A or retinol:	Required for the maintenance and functioning of epithelial tissues, especially cells which synthesize glycoproteins; normal epithelial tissues in eyes, bones, nerves, skin, glands, and mucous membranes attest to the functions of the vitamin
Vitamin D:	Promotes intestinal absorption of calcium and perhaps phosphorus and their utilization in ossification of bones and teeth
Vitamin E:	A lipid antioxidant prevents formation of peroxides from polyunsaturated fatty acids
Ascorbic Acid:	Related to formation of collagen from hydroxyproline by addition of hydroxyl group to proline; collagen is an intercellular substance which maintains tissue structure including strength of capillary wall, bone structure and other tissues
Thiamine:	Requirement related to calorie intake (0.4 mg/1000 Cal) and increases with increase in dietary carbohydrate; functions as a cocarboxylase in degradation during intermediary carbohydrate metabolism; pyruvic acid accumulates in toxic levels during deficiency
Riboflavin:	Requirement related to calorie intake (0.7 mg/100 Cal) and increases with increase in dietary fat; functions in a molecule as a dehydrogenase in energy metabolism
Niacin:	Related to tryptophan, an essential amino acid, 1 mg niacin is equivalent to 60 mg tryptophan. Related to fat metabolism as a dehydrogenase; massive doses (100 mg and larger) are effective in lowering serum cholesterol levels and in improving circulation by dialating periferal capillaries
Cobalamin:	This extrinsic factor is required to cure pernicious anemia but depends on the intrinsic factor in gastric mucosa which is needed for absorption of cobalamin from ingested food
Pyridoxine:	The phosphorylated molecule functions as an enzyme in synthesis and/or catabolism of all amino acids as well as in interconversion of glycine and serine and of the formation of cysteine from methionine

excess amounts. Such a test consists of these steps:

1. A known amount of a vitamin is given to a person in a postabsorptive state (12 hours since last food intake).
2. The amount excreted in the next several urinations is determined during specified time intervals up to about six hours.
3. The percentage excreted is indicative of tissue saturation:
   (a) *a high percentage excretion* indicates that the tissues were saturated and could absorb only limited additional amounts,
   (b) *a low percentage excretion* indicates that the tissues were depleted

and therefore absorbed additional amounts; naturally all levels of saturation can exist.

The human body like that of all animals is a coordinated mechanism completely integrated and not an arrangement of separate entities, organs, or processes. This whole body needs all the nutrients simultaneously and continuously; the amount is dependent on the rate of metabolism. It has facilities for short-term pools, depots or even storage sites depending on the chemical nature of the nutrients. In general, a regular supply of these nutrients is needed in the diet at intervals throughout the day; reserves of water soluble nutrients are sufficient for only a limited period of hours. The liver serves as a depot for all vitamins, however, the blood level both in cells and plasma is generally indicative of the supply available to the cells.

Fat soluble vitamins can be stored in concentrations which require consumption of these vitamins only several times a week to assure adequacy of intake. Excessive amounts of vitamin D may be consumed from fortified foods by people who have no special need for vitamin D. The need for vitamin D has been established only for certain times in life such as growth, pregnancy, or lactation.

Symptoms of vitamin deficiencies are rare, mostly because marginal diets are not deficient in vitamins alone. (Table 9.4 lists a few clinical symptoms of some of the vitamins.) Thus in most cases, dietary deficiencies are multiple in nature and may be referred to as a *malnutrition syndrome*. However, since vitamins A and C are rather unique and limited in their dietary sources, either or both of these are often supplied in inadequate amounts according to dietary surveys. Since ascorbic acid is water soluble and chemically unstable in many procedures practiced in the home kitchen and in commercial food production, it is the one most apt to be deficient.

Pharmaceutical companies are generous to supply information and pictures of laboratory animals and of human beings with various typical deficiency symptoms. In general, these symptoms are often described as lassitude, weakness, anorexia, anemia, edema, vague pains in muscles and joints, dermatitis, poor quality hair, and mental dullness. However, lack of the common vitamins produces deficiency symptoms which are easily identified.

Interpretation of Recommended Dietary Allowances (RDA)

The Recommended Dietary Allowances (RDA) are based on levels required to prevent symptoms of deficiency plus a "margin for safety." This "margin for safety" takes into account two major areas which cause

Table 9.4   Clinical symptoms of vitamin deficiencies.

Vitamins of Dietary Significance	Clinical Symptoms of Deficiency
Vitamin A or retinol:	Dry, itchy, irritated epithelial tissues, which include mucous linings of respiratory, gastro-intestinal, and urogenital tracts; the skin develops spines in sebaceous glands and hair follicles; high incidence of abortion and fetal death; frequent and severe infections especially of respiratory tract
Vitamin D:	None until bone changes occur in the epiphyses with painfully swollen joints, delayed closure of fontanel in the skull of infants, delayed dentition, etc., malalignment of leg bones, malocclusion of teeth
Vitamin E:	Wide variety of symptoms in various animals, thus far symptoms are nonspecific in people
Ascorbic Acid:	Capillary fragility leads to gums with red swollen spots which may bleed without apparent cause; skin bruises which show multiple petechae; vague pains in swollen joints and muscles; more frequent and severe infections; loosened teeth; beading and fracture of ribs involved in rachitic scurvy
Thiamine:	Deficiency leads to elevation of pyruvic acid levels in blood which results in abnormal neuromuscular responses in reflexes, "foot drop syndrome" and other phenomena including anorexia and gastro-intestinal atony leading to constipation
Riboflavin:	Skin lesions (cheilosis) develop first at corners of mouth at the mucosal-epidermal junction. Photophobia and vascular proliferation into the cornea of the eye associated with itching and burning sensation; congenital deformities related to cleft palate, club feet, and leg malformations
Cobalamin:	Development of syndrome of glossitis, anemia, and neurological changes; macrocytic anemia responds only to intravenous injection of cobalamin
Pyridoxine:	Appears to lower antibody production by reducing synthesis of nucleic acids required for antibody and immune protein synthesis

variations; namely, variation in the food as actually consumed by people and variation in the absorption and in the physiological need of a person for a given vitamin on a specific day. Variation in nutrient composition of food goes back to its production — the species, the cultivation, climate, harvest, handling, processing, and storage methods prior to reaching the retail market for purchase by the consumer. The final variation in the vitamin content of a food depends on manipulation and treatment inflicted on the food in the kitchen at home; the final variation is caused by the diner and his selectivity in eating. Thus the statement "many a slip

Table 9.5 Comparison of the requirements for the fat soluble vitamins per kilogram of body weight, RDA, revised 1968.

	Age	Wt.	Fat Soluble Vitamins		
			Vit. A	Vit. D	Vit. E
	yr	kg	IU	IU	IU
Infants	0–⅙	4	375	100	1.3
	⅙–½	7	214	57	0.7
	½–1	9	167	44	0.6
Children	1–2	12	167	33	0.8
	2–3	14	143	29	0.7
	3–4	16	151	25	0.6
	4 6	19	132	21	0.5
	6–8	23	152	17	0.7
	8–10	28	125	14	0.5
Males	10–12	35	129	11	0.6
	12–14	43	116	9	0.5
	14–18	59	85	7	0.4
	18–22	67	75	6	0.5
	22–35	70	71	—	0.4
	35–55	70	71	—	0.4
	55–75+	70	71	—	0.4
Females	10–12	35	129	11	0.6
	12–14	44	114	9	0.5
	14–16	52	96	8	0.5
	16–18	54	93	7	0.5
	18–22	58	86	7	0.4
	22–35	58	86	—	0.4
	35–55	58	86	—	0.4
	55–75+	58	86	—	0.4
Pregnancy		65*	92	6	0.5
Lactation		60*	133	7	0.5

*Approximate figures.

between the cup and the lip" typifies the multiplicity of factors to affect composition of food as it is actually eaten.

The individual person has variation in the absorption of vitamins related to the total composition of the diet, to certain environmental factors related to eating, and the health of the gastro-intestinal tract at that time. Fiber content of the diet, motility of the gastro-intestinal tract, emotional state, and other components are factors which affect

Table 9.6   Recommended daily vitamin intakes for age intervals, NRC's 1968 revision

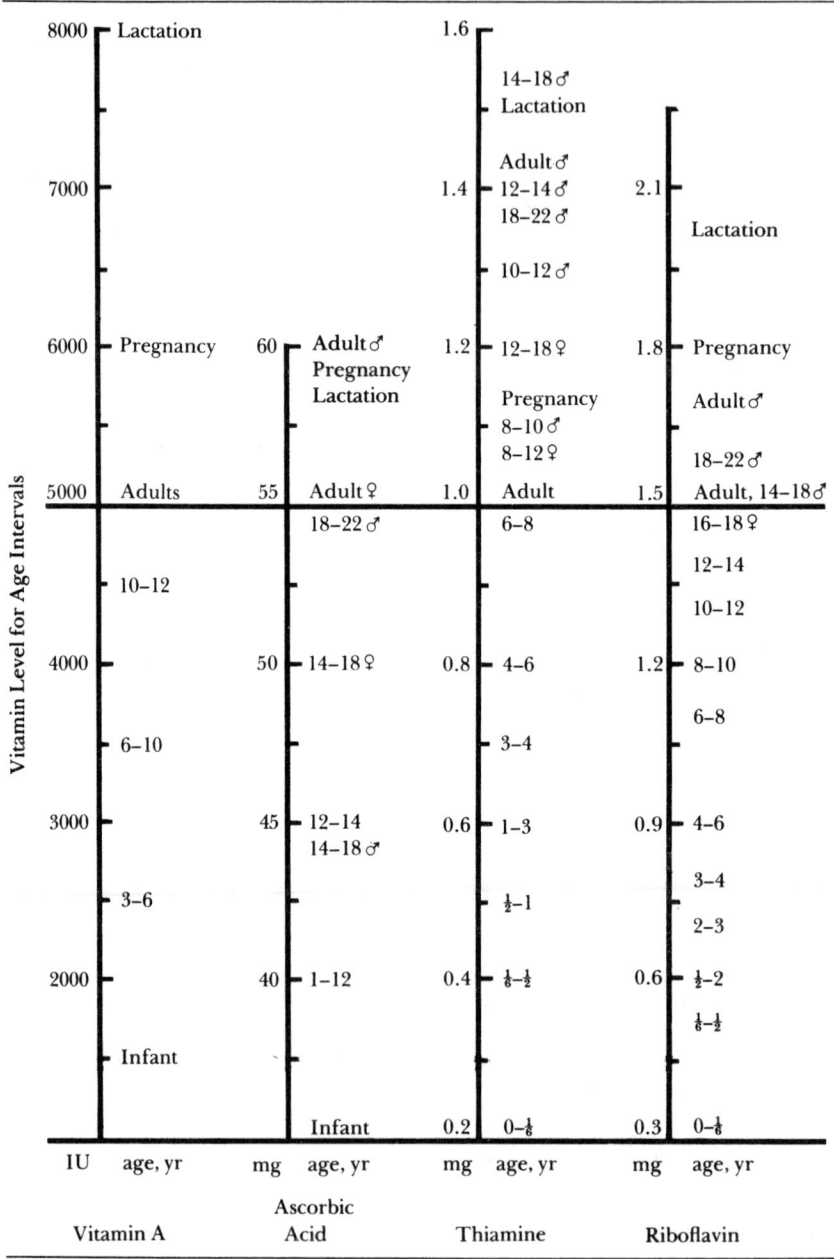

Vitamin Level for Age Intervals

	Vitamin A			Ascorbic Acid			Thiamine			Riboflavin
8000	Lactation		1.6							
						14–18 ♂ Lactation				
7000			1.4			Adult ♂ 12–14 ♂ 18–22 ♂	2.1	Lactation		
						10–12 ♂				
6000	Pregnancy	60	Adult ♂ Pregnancy Lactation	1.2	12–18 ♀	Pregnancy 8–10 ♂ 8–12 ♀	1.8	Pregnancy Adult ♂ 18–22 ♂		
5000	Adults	55	Adult ♀	1.0	Adult	1.5	Adult, 14–18 ♂			
			18–22 ♂		6–8		16–18 ♀			
	10–12						12–14			
							10–12			
4000		50	14–18 ♀	0.8	4–6	1.2	8–10			
	6–10				3–4		6–8			
3000		45	12–14 14–18 ♂	0.6	1–3	0.9	4–6			
	3–6				½–1		3–4 2–3			
2000		40	1–12	0.4	⅙–½	0.6	½–2 ⅙–½			
	Infant									
			Infant	0.2	0–⅙	0.3	0–⅙			
IU	age, yr	mg	age, yr	mg	age, yr	mg	age, yr			

absorption in people. The vitamin need of specific tissues is affected by the rate of catabolic and anabolic activity which is related to activity, age, sex, rate of growth, and health. Any infection and fever increases catabolism of vitamins, therefore, the need for an increased dietary supply of vitamins for the duration of the infection and fever. Stressful situations which include pregnancy, lactation, surgery, and other periods of stress also increase the need for an increased supply of vitamins.

Since dietaries are usually planned for the food a person is to consume in a day and the amounts eaten are dependent on the appetite and taste preferences of the individual, seldom is the dietary need for vitamins considered on the basis of body size. A mother or even a dietitian has difficulty in visualizing that the dietary needs per kilogram of body size are highest for the newborn infant and lowest for the adult. Table 9.5 interprets the RDA for fat soluble vitamins as quantities per kilogram of body weight for the various ages of both sexes. The data warrant consideration in dietary planning since quantities recommended for the vitamins decrease with increase in age. Table 9.6 interprets the RDA for the vitamins in a modified bar graph to show the relative daily intake recommended for the various age groups. Such analysis should help to develop a visual image of the nutrients to be supplied in daily dietary designs.

Therapeutic Dosages

The RDA specifies the amounts of vitamins required to maintain the person at various ages, sex and when pregnant or lactating. However, if a deficiency should have been diagnosed, the quantity of each vitamin required to reestablish health is greatly increased. If the need is only moderate and no digestive disturbance is involved, the therapeutic dose can be given by mouth; if the deficiency is severe, has been of longer duration, and gastro-intestinal impairment is suspected (or even proved), the dosage must be supplied parenterally. Generalizations specifying the amounts of therapeutic vitamins are not generally published, but students should be aware of the massive dosages that are recommended.

Activities for Student Learning

1. Review previous readings from sociology, anthropology, history, medicine, or historical novels and note reference to abnormal physical characteristics of people who could have had symptoms of vitamin deficiencies.

2. Study additional information on vitamins published in suitable reference sources.
3. Analyze empirical chemical structures of some of the vitamins, note their complexity, and the arrangement of elements as related to function; also note the different chemical forms in which some vitamins occur.
4. View a film or slides showing dietary deficiencies of the vitamins such as *Vitamin Deficiencies* by Lederele Laboratories.
5. For students to develop skill in group and individual instruction:
   (a) Role-play a teaching situation stressing the physiological characteristics of the two groups of vitamins.
   (b) Divide the class into competition groups to plan games which will facilitate learning about the functions, cellular involvements, symptoms of deficiencies and needs for the major vitamins.
   (c) Prepare and present a talk for a particular lay group in your community on the "Therapeutic Daily Dosage of Vitamins."

6. *Hot Tips:*

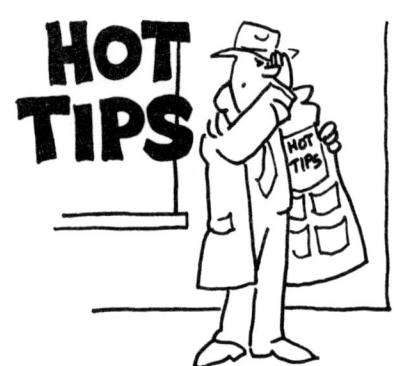

New Words:

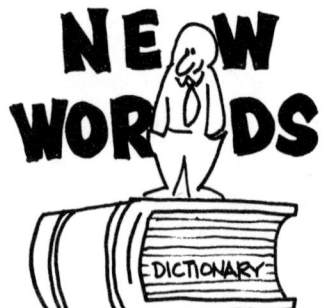

SOURCES OF VITAMINS

Objectives

1. To identify from food composition tables those foods which are the most concentrated sources of each vitamin.
2. To plan and evaluate menus for specific families from different cultural eating patterns and food expenditures that will meet the dietary needs of the family involved.
3. To demonstrate the relationship of recommended food preparation procedures as they are related to vitamin retention and supply in diets.

Dietary Levels of Vitamins in Households in the United States

Table 9.7 gives a clear picture of sources of nutrients that people actually consume and the percentages of the common vitamins supplied by different food groups in regular family diets. This in turn demonstrates the dietary disaster which occurs when a food group is omitted or consumed in minimal amounts. About half of the dietary supply for vitamin A is derived from Fruits and Vegetables Groups in addition to 85% of vitamin C. Along with these generous amounts of vitamins, vegetables and fruit supply a low level of energy or calories. On the other hand, the percentages of nutrients furnished by Cereal and Grain Products are 25 of the calories, 40 of thiamine, almost 20 of riboflavin, and 20–25 of niacin. The riboflavin supply was derived mostly from Dairy Products (almost 40%) and Cereal Products (about 20%). Analyses show that without either of these two very important food groups, a serious deficiency can occur in the B vitamins of family diets.

Two food groups usurp about 60–65% of the food dollar, namely, Meats and other Protein Foods and Miscellaneous. The Meats and other Protein Foods also supply from one-fourth to one-third of all the vitamins except ascorbic acid. Too bad that the 17+% of the food dollar spent for Miscellaneous items furnishes only energy or calories and modest amounts of niacin (17%).

Regionally in the United States only slight variations occur in the percentage of vitamins furnished by each food group. The USDA publication of *Dietary Levels of Households* gives data for different areas of residence, employment and income level which show some variation in nutrients supplied in the various dietary patterns of families. These differences are not reflected by mean values for regions.

This survey offers guidance to people for evaluation of the necessity for dietary improvement perhaps through the use of concentrated

Table 9.7 Money value, energy, and vitamins by food group and region: USDA Household Food Consumption Survey Reports 6, 7, 8, 9, and 10, 1965–66.

Food Group & Region	Percentage of Total Food						
	Money value	Food energy	Vit. A	Thiamine	Riboflavin	Niacin	Ascorbic acid
I. *Dairy Products*							
North east	12.8	13.7	12.5	10.7	39.1	2.4	5.0
North central	12.6	13.5	13.9	10.8	39.4	2.4	5.6
South	12.4	11.0	11.3	9.2	35.7	2.2	5.2
West	12.6	13.5	11.9	11.2	39.5	2.6	5.4
U.S.	12.6	12.7	12.5	10.3	38.2	2.4	5.3
II. *Protein Foods*							
North east	38.5	27.0	24.3	28.4	29.6	44.1	1.0
North central	38.2	28.6	23.6	31.2	30.4	43.6	1.0
South	38.0	27.2	24.8	28.8	30.3	41.8	0.4
West	36.7	28.8	22.9	28.9	30.5	44.9	1.1
U.S.	37.9	27.8	20.1	29.4	30.2	43.4	1.1
III. *Vegetables*							
North east	11.3	6.0	42.0	13.0	6.6	11.8	37.4
North central	12.3	6.2	40.3	12.3	6.3	11.9	38.6
South	12.9	5.0	44.1	11.8	7.1	10.9	47.3
West	12.1	5.5	44.1	12.5	6.7	11.2	39.2
U.S.	12.2	5.7	42.5	12.4	6.7	11.5	40.9
IV. *Fruits*							
North east	7.5	4.2	7.3	7.8	2.8	3.1	50.4
North central	7.5	4.0	7.1	6.5	2.7	2.9	48.1
South	6.7	3.1	7.1	5.1	2.3	2.5	41.8
West	8.5	4.4	8.4	7.2	2.9	3.3	49.1
U.S.	7.4	3.8	7.3	6.4	2.6	2.9	47.0
V. *Grain Products*							
North east	12.5	25.5	1.6	38.0	17.5	20.9	0.9
North central	12.2	24.4	1.5	37.4	17.6	20.6	1.0
South	12.4	27.1	1.4	43.7	21.6	26.3	0.6
West	12.2	24.5	1.3	39.1	17.1	21.1	1.1
U.S.	12.3	25.6	2.4	39.9	18.8	22.5	0.9
VI. *Miscellaneous*							
North east	17.3	23.5	12.2	2.0	4.3	17.6	5.4
North central	17.2	23.3	13.5	1.7	3.7	18.5	5.6
South	17.7	36.7	11.3	1.3	3.0	16.3	3.9
West	17.9	23.2	11.3	1.3	3.1	16.9	4.1
U.S.	17.5	24.4	12.1	1.3	3.5	17.3	4.8

food sources or dietary supplements. For example, those households which do not consume regular amounts of fruits definitely will have an ascorbic acid deficiency. In this case, the need for dietary improvement or for food which is a concentrated source of ascorbic acid is apparent. Interpretation of the cause for omission of a food group should be included in all dietary surveys. The individual homemaker should think about why she failed to supply a food group in her dietary design for her household. Such a self-analysis to identify "a moment of truth" is crucial in nutrition education. It assists a homemaker to identify her motives in feeding the family and to realize that food has a physiological function in addition to satisfying hunger.

Those who hope to enjoy the benefits of adequate nutrition and optimum vitamin intake need to design their dietary routines to include at each meal some food sources of the B vitamins and of ascorbic acid. Once daily or multiweekly intake of the fat soluble vitamins is considered sufficient if the mean daily intake equals the RDA for that vitamin.

Analysis of Pharmaceutical Sources of Vitamins

When the intake of fat soluble vitamins reaches levels that are ten or more times the RDA for an extended period of time, symptoms of toxicity may be identified and even death can result. The RDA of 5000 IU of vitamin A as carotene and retinol is generous and allows for a "margin of safety." Therapeutic dosage, which may be as high as 200,000 IU daily, should be restricted to a relatively limited period of time, e.g., two weeks. No evidence supports the myth that "if a little bit is good, a lot is better," but rather research shows that "enough of a good thing is enough." Toxic levels of vitamin D are being given to young children by overzealous, uninformed mothers. The American Medical Association and other health-oriented organizations have cautioned against excessive vitamin intake. Few foods, even when eaten in gluttonous amounts, have sufficient vitamin concentration to be toxic. The exceptions are livers from polar bear, seals, and other marine animals which have been reported to contain 13,000–18,000 IU per gram in contrast to calf's liver containing 225 IU per gram. Deaths have been attributed to consumption of excessive amounts of polar bear liver with the vitamin A value listed as the toxic substance.

The advent of synthetic vitamins has made vitamins available in simple sugar coated pills at any grocery or drug store; their promotion by high pressure advertising has encouraged people to seek comfort and relief in vitamin therapy whether needed or not. Suggested adverse effects have been reported from massive dosage of some vitamins consumed over a period of time. The harm has been also to the purse and economy of household budgets. Furthermore, at times the well-meaning home-maker has gained false comfort from substituting a vitamin pill for a balanced diet; a vitamin pill has enabled children to be allowed to suffer malnutrition resulting from minimal and irregular intakes of protein, mineral, and even energy-giving nutrients. Thus intakes of even harm-less amounts of vitamins in pills or tablets may be detrimental to child growth and development when these are substituted for an adequate nutrient intake served in regular balanced meals.

Another concern which confronts the shopper and consumer of pharmaceutical vitamins is represented by the variety of products avail-able from which she has to make a selection. See Table 9.8 for a com-parison between only four of the different brands that are currently available on the retail market. The decision has to be made as to whether to buy a single vitamin like thiamine or whether to buy a multiple vitamin product, i.e., one which contains either nine or fifteen vitamins, or even one which supplies in addition to all the vitamins, a variety of mineral

Table 9.8   Comparison of selected available vitamin tablets.

Vitamin	Unit	Multiple Vitamin Tablets Brand 1	Brand 2	Therapeutic Vitamin Tablets Brand 1	Brand 2
A	IU	5000	5000	25,000	25,000
D	IU	400	400	400	400
C	mg	50	50	200	200
E	IU	—	—	15	15
Thiamine	mg	2	2	10	10
Riboflavin	mg	2.5	2.5	5.0	5.0
Niacinamide	mg	20	20	100	100
Pyridoxine	mg	1	1	50	50
Cobalamin	mcg	1	1	5	5
Calcium panthonate	mg	1	1	20	—
Copper	mg	—	—	—	2
Iron	mg	—	—	—	20
Magnesium	mg	—	—	—	75
Manganese	mg	—	—	—	1
Zinc	mg	—	—	—	1.5
Price per 100 tablets		$2.98	$0.99	$7.95	$6.49

elements and maybe other compounds. Even this is not all, but the confused consumer needs to decide if an obscure brand at 99 cents per 100 tablets is as good as a highly advertized brand at $2.98 per 100 tablets with the label listing the same quantity of the same vitamins. Furthermore, should the consumer choose a multivitamin tablet in which the concentrations resemble the amount specified by the RDA or would a "Therapeutic formula" type tablet be better when the amounts are from five to ten times those needed daily? An analysis of the variety of vitamin preparations available without prescription adds to the confusion in trying to decide on tablets to swallow whole, chewable ones, drops, or even a vitamin tonic which is also rich in alcohol. That such decisions face the consumer is obvious when one studies the comparison of four different brands of vitamins in Table 9.8.

Finally, should the consumer "ditch the whole thing" and find comfort in organic gardening? Maybe what the tired housewife, the teenagers with tired blood, and the husband and father with a threatening ulcer really need is quiet, uninterrupted rest instead of vitamin pills, mineral compounds, or tonics. Nonetheless, when vitamin concentrates are needed according to diagnosis made by a qualified doctor, pharmaceutical sources may be a real life saver.

Activities for Student Learning

1. Choose a book on sociology, anthropology, history, medicine, or an historical novel and note the role which food and eating occupied in the lives of people and the events around them. Observe the sources of vitamins in the eating habits of these people, their methods of food preparation which retained vitamins in food, and those that contributed to decreases in vitamin content.
2. Refer to "Nutrient Content of Food" in Unit 4 and other references in order to prepare a chart showing how the chemical properties of vitamins relate to their retention in food:

Vitamin	Chemical Reactivity	Recommended Procedures in Food Preparation

3. Starting with a pint of milk and a serving (3 or 4 oz EP) of meat, plan the amounts of other foods required to meet the day's allowance of vitamins.
4. People need to be familiar with pharmaceutical sources of nutrients, especially with vitamins and mineral-vitamin preparations which are a massive portion of the drug industry in the United States.

Their sales promotion sponsors a multimillion dollar business encouraging American mothers to rely on vitamin pills to compensate for any dietary deficiency.

Analyze some of the popular brands that are available to the consumer by completing the following:

Dietary Supplements: pharmaceutical vitamins

Brand	Dosage and cost/day	Nutrient content and concentration per capsule

References and Suggested Readings

Ariaey-Nejad, *et al.* Thiamin metabolism in man, *Amer. J. Clin. Nutr.*, **23**: 764 (1970).

Bailey, D. A., *et al.* Vitamin C supplementation related to physiological response to exercise in smoking and nonsmoking subjects, *Amer. J. Clin. Nutr.*, **23**: 905 (1970).

Campbell, J. A. Dietary factors affecting vitamin requirements, *Proc. Nutr. Soc.*, **23**, 31 (1964).

Campbell, J. A., and Morrison, A. B. Some factors affecting absorption of vitamins, *Amer. J. Clin. Nutr.*, **12**, 162 (1963).

Council on food & nutrition, general policy on addition of specific nutrients to foods, *J. AMA*, **178**, 1024 (1961).

Darby, W. J. Scurvy developing during therapy for psychoneurosis, *Nutr. Today*, **1**: 3, 20 (1966).

Davis, T. R. A., Gershoff, S. N., and Gamble, D. F. Review of studies of vitamin and mineral nutrition in the United States (1950–1968), *J. Nutr. Educ.*, **1**: 2, Suppl. 1, 41 (1969).

DeLuca, H. F., and Suttie, J. W., (eds.) *The Fat Soluble Vitamins.* New York: Amer. Univ. Press, 1970.

Gershoff, S. N. Effects of dietary levels of macronutrients on vitamin requirements, *Federation Proc.*, **23**, 1077 (1964).

Gyorgy, P., and Pearson, W. N. *The Vitamins*, 2nd ed., Vols. VI & VII. New York: Academic Press, 1967.

Hardinge, M. G., and Crooks, H. Lesser known vitamins in foods, *J. Amer. Dietet. Assoc.*, **38**, 240 (1961).

Hodges, R. E. The effect of stress on ascorbic acid metabolism in man, *Nutr. Today*, **5**: 1, 11 (1970).

King, C. G. Practical and novel advances in relation to vitamin C, *J. Nutr. Educ.*, **1**, 16 (1969).

Morton, H. A. *Fat-soluble Vitamins.* New York: Pergamon, 1971.

National Academy of Sciences. Recommended Dietary Allowances. 7th ed., Publication No. 1964, Washington, D.C., 1968.

Olson, R. E. Mode of action of vitamin K, *Nutr. Rev.*, **28**: 171, 1970.

Osifo, B. O. A. Effect of folic acid and iron in the prevention of nutritional anaemias in pregnancy in Nigeria, *Brit. J. Nutr.*, **24**: 689 (1970).

Pelletier, O. Cigarette smoking and vitamin C, *Nutr. Today*, **5**: 3, 12 (1970).

Phillips, D. C. Three-dimensional structure of an enzyme molecule, *Scientific American* *215*, No. 5: 78 (1966).

Present Knowledge in Nutrition. New York: The Nutrition Foundation, 1967.

Review of studies of vitamin and mineral nutrition in the United States (1950–1968), *J. Nutr. Educ.*, **1**, 2, Suppl. 1 (1969).

Rivlin, R. S. Riboflavin metabolism, *New Eng. J. Med.*, **283**: 463–472 (1970).

Robinson, F. A. *The Vitamin Co-Factors of Enzyme Systems.* New York: Pergamon, 1966.

Roe, D. A. Nutrient toxicity with excessive intake I. vitamins, *N.Y. J. Med.*, **66**: 869 (1966).

Ross, R. Wound healing, *Scientific American 220*, No. 6: 40 (1969).

Schwartz, P. L. Ascorbic acid in wound healing – a review. *J.A.D.A.*, **56**: 497 (1970).

Sebrell, W. H., and Harris, R. S. *The Vitamins*, 2nd ed., Vols. I & II. New York: Academic Press, 1967–68.

Symposium: Advances in the detection of nutrition deficiencies in man, *Amer. J. Clin. Nutr.*, 20 (June 1967).

U.S.D.A. – Conserving the Nutritive Values in Foods, Home and Garden Bulletin No. 90, U.S. Govt. Ptg. Office, Washington, D.C., 1963.

Vitamin Manual. Kalamazoo, Mich.: Upjohn, 1963.

Vitler, R. W. Vitamins, minerals, and anemia, *J. AMA*, **175**, 152 (1961).

Wagner, A. F., and Foikers, K. *Vitamins and Coenzymes.* New York: Interscience, 1964.

INVENTORY OF KNOWLEDGE

Part I

You should be able to match the name of one vitamin listed on the right with each of the statements and record its letter in the space provided.

_____ 1. Related to irradiation of skin by the sun

_____ 2. Concentration related to acidity in fruits

_____ 3. Related to tryptophan conversion

_____ 4. Diets of the early English sailor were often deficient

_____ 5. Affects normal appetite

_____ 6. Pure vitamin is deep yellow color

_____ 7. Early symptom of deficiency is dermatitis

_____ 8. Dietary supplement will not cure pernicious anemia

_____ 9. Liver is *not* a reliable source

_____10. Aids in proper calcification of teeth

_____11. Pellagra preventative factor

_____12. One of the first vitamins to be chemically synthesized

_____13. Phosphorus and calcium are important in its function

_____14. Intakes in excess of 25,000 units may become toxic

(a) Vitamin A
(b) Ascorbic Acid
(c) Niacin
(d) Riboflavin
(e) Vitamin D
(f) Thiamine
(g) Cobalamin

_____15. Apt to be deficient in diets of nondairy food consumers

_____16. Correctly called "retinal" as its legal term

_____17. Is identified as irradiated ergosterol

_____18. Symptoms include condition called cheilosis

_____19. Contains the element sulfur in its chemical makeup

_____20. Most easily decomposed of all vitamins

_____21. Deficient in diets which consist of mostly cooked foods

_____22. Dietary supply reduced by use of nonfat dry milk products instead of whole milk ones

_____23. U.S.'s RDA is very high in comparison to standards used by other countries

_____24. Involved in neuromuscular functions

_____25. Car accidents at night may be related to night blindness

Part II

Answer these questions in concise statements:

26. What events or practices lead to the discovery of the first vitamins?

27. What are the general functions of the vitamins?

28. What are the major causes of reduction of the original vitamin content in food?

29. What is the basis on which to decide which vitamin supplement should be selected?

10

The Concern of the Consumer for Food and Nutrition

How Should Nutrition be Related to Consumer Education?

The extensive nutrition research and increased governmental regulations together with the many publications, lectures, and classes in nutrition of this country cannot guarantee that its people are well nourished. In the final analysis, the consumer has the freedom to choose the food he eats and is responsible for his own nutrition and nutritional status. The consumer's responsibility is shared to some extent by the individual who selects the food and plans, prepares, and serves the meals for other people, both adults and children. This may be a homemaker, mother, dietitian, school lunch manager, home economist in business, teacher, restaurateur, or the proprietor of a burger-bar. All of them assume some responsibility for the nutrition and subsequently the health of the people they serve. Good nutritional status of people requires that those who serve food to the consumer as well as the consumer himself, select food first for its nutritive value and in addition for whatever other reasons influence his food choices.

Education for the consumer is inadequate unless it provides an understanding of nutrition. Many of the common guidelines for food buying which stress the importance of sanitation, appearance, freshness, grade labeling, wholesomeness, quality control, and thrift do not necessarily assure any nutritional value. Fresh raw produce and properly processed and stored food as well as solid pack food tend to contain more nutrients than those that are wilted, overexposed to heat and air, or canned in a watery pack. Their superior nutritive quality is seldom the major concern of the processor, seller, or even of the consumer. Too often the consumer forgets that the ultimate value of any food is the quality and quantity of its nutrient content. Only when adequate nutritive value is combined with wholesomeness, palatability, and a reasonable price, does the food buyer get his money's worth.

As a citizen the consumer has the responsibility of being actively concerned that the nutritive quality of food is the primary goal of the food production, processing, and marketing industry, of government and private consumer protection agencies, and, most of all, of the consumer himself in his food selection and eating habits.

PROBLEMS FACING THE CONSUMER OF FOOD

Objectives
1. To identify the efforts which are made to assure the safety and wholesomeness of the food supply.
2. To list major problems on consumer choice and purchase of food.
3. To identify each individual's own responsibility for his success as a food consumer.

The Situation of Today

A trip to the supermarket causes today's consumer to marvel at the thousands of foods displayed. Was he tempted to buy or did he hesitate and wonder about their quality and nutrient content? Did he enjoy the hamburger and ice cream at the drive-in or did he worry about their ingredients, cleanliness, and safety? The majority of people in this country buys and eats food freely at any regular food outlet whether it be a supermarket, roadside stand, drive-in, restaurant, or tearoom with little or no thought about the nutrient content, wholesomeness, and safety of the food. Generally such faith seems justified. Application of science and technology to the production and distribution of food has assured the United States consumer a superabundance and almost unlimited variety of generally wholesome and palatable food. Moreover, food prices have advanced less than prices of most other goods and services, while incomes have increased. From 1957–59 to the first half of 1968, incomes rose 63% and food expenditures 37%. According to Gale (1971), the consumer expenditure for food in 1960 averaged 20% of his disposable income. In 1969 and in 1970, this expenditure had decreased to 16.7% as an overall average. Thus the principle that "As incomes increase, the percentage spent for food decreases" is evident, although other factors also influence cost of food expenditures.

Is the consumer aware of the power he wields in the food industry when he makes his choices in the food market? Consumers in the aggregate determine through patronage, or the lack of it, which business firms succeed and which fail. They decide the kind, variety, and quality of foods that remain on the market through their response to how they are advertised, promoted, and sold, and to some extent their price. Every dollar the consumer spends acts as a vote in favor of the purpose for which it was used. Moreover, the consumer in this country has not only freedom of choice in the use of much of his money income but also the opportunity, in fact the responsibility, to express an opinion to both business personnel and government officials with regard to the kind of foods, services, and regulations he wants or does not want. When consumers do this with reasoning and in large enough numbers, their wishes will be heeded by both the food industry and the government.

Since the 1940s a revolution of changes has occurred in all segments of the food industry. These present both benefits and problems to the food buyer and consumer. Scientific and technological developments in production and distribution have introduced hundreds of new food products, including imitation foods such as simulated meat. Prepackaging of foods in a large number and variety of containers, which are now used on 85% of the foods on the market, makes it difficult or impossible for the consumer to examine what he is buying. Moreover, many labels do not provide adequate information for intelligent choices. Fractional amounts of content complicate price comparisons. The number and variety of convenience foods are increasing. Basic to many of these new products is the increasing use of multiple ingredients and of additives in food processing. Further complicating the possible quality of food is the increasing pollution of air, water, and land including the dangers of atomic fallout, industrial waste, pesticides, fertilizers, and human waste. In addition, mass production and distribution have separated the producer from the consumer and made consumer-retailer relations casual and impersonal. Thus consumer choices are more complex and the ability to evaluate food selections on the market more difficult. Even the educated consumer may not understand the significance of the long list of chemical terms on many food packages. Recent widely publicized negative news about food, such as the danger of cyclamates and the questionable quality of sausages or ham, caused consumer uneasiness and stimulated a desire for more government protection. Judging by the large number of Federal and state government regulations concerned with food, some desire for governmental protection has existed for a number of years.

GOVERNMENTAL PROTECTION OF THE FOOD CONSUMER

Objectives

1. To list the reasons for government involvement in protection of the consumer.
2. To identify the responsibility for consumer well-being currently assigned to various Federal governmental agencies.
3. To identify examples of compliance with regulations concerning food.

Federal Agencies Concerned With Consumer Protection

History shows that government regulations in the food industry are not new; a Sanskrit law of 300 B.C. imposed fines on those who sold adulterated grains and oils. In the United States the first food law which "penalized the seller of diseased, corrupted, or unwholesome provisions" was passed in Massachusetts in 1784. Federal government action in consumer protection has accelerated since President John F. Kennedy, the first president to devote a message to Congress on consumer welfare, proclaimed these four rights of the consumer:

1. The right to safety. The consumer can feel secure that goods and services on the market will not endanger his health when used as directed.
2. The right to be informed. He can readily get adequate, reliable information essential to making intelligent decisions in the use of his money for the purchase of goods and services and their use.
3. The right to be heard. He has the opportunity to be heard in

government on an equal basis with business and other interests.
4. The right to choose. He can make his own choices without pressure from others.

Since the promulgation of these rights, many individuals and groups, private and public, have tried to influence governmental action on Federal, state, and local levels with various results and achievements. Troelstrup in the 1970 revision of his consumer education textbook described the Federal Consumer Program in these words:

> ... legislation and executive action in the name of the consumer protection has produced a sprawling, uncoordinated maze of laws and agencies frequently working at cross purposes and usually cursed by a too-little-too-late timidity. Thus consumer interests have not been served.

A comprehensive study in 1961 of the Consumer Protection Activities of the Federal Departments and Agencies reported that 33 of the 35 major departments and agencies were involved in some kind of consumer activity, but that of the 296 activities listed by them, only 103 dealt directly with consumer protection. At the same time, only one million dollars of the vast Federal budget was used for these agencies. Their major effort in the consumer interest was against fraud and deception and for the enforcement of laws against the sale of adulterated and unsafe food and drugs. Because of the fragmentation of legal protection among different areas of the government, the diversity and detail of many of the acts, and the many changes that are being made currently, the total program is difficult to describe clearly and accurately.

In general, consumer protection in food means protection against economic cheats, i.e., spending money with little value received as the result of fraudulent practices,

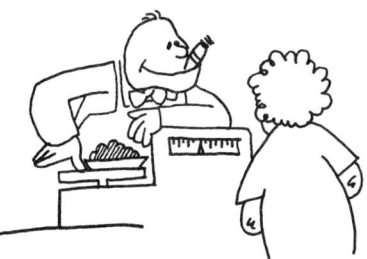

Fig. 10.1 Consumer protection in food means protection against the economic cheat.

and against unwholesome and unsafe products which endanger the health of the user. On the Federal level in 1971 the major agencies concerned with food were:

1. The Food and Drug Administration (FDA) and U.S. Public Health Service in the Department of Health, Education, and Welfare (HEW).

2. The U.S. Department of Agriculture (USDA).
3. The Bureau of Standards in the Department of Commerce.
4. The Federal Trade Commission (FTC).
5. Office of Consumer Affairs, Executive Office of the President.
6. Miscellaneous agencies.

None of these agencies devotes all of its efforts to food and nutrition though each makes some contribution directly and/or indirectly. Generally the Federal agencies are concerned with food in interstate (among states) commerce, whereas state agencies are concerned with food produced and sold within the state (intrastate commerce), although the Wholesome Meat Act of 1967 and the Wholesome Poultry Products Act of 1968 have changed this concept to some extent.

Major agencies in the state are usually the State Health Department in charge of food and drugs and State Department of Agriculture in charge of meats, poultry, fruits, vegetables, and usually weights and measures. Because of significant variations among the state programs for consumer protection, only the Federal programs are included in this brief presentation. Individuals who need detailed and complete information should obtain the most recent releases from the state or Federal agency.

The Food and Drug Administration (FDA) in U.S. Department of Health, Education, and Welfare (HEW)

The FDA, established in 1927, is the largest single agency devoted entirely to consumer protection. Although food, including nonalcoholic beverages, drugs, cosmetics, therapeutic devices, and safety aspects of some other products in interstate commerce are under its jurisdiction, only food is included in this discussion.

The overall responsibilities of the FDA in the area of food and nutrition may be summarized as follows:

A. Setting of standards of identity, quality, fill of container, and enrichment of foods:

1. Standards of identity or definition: these establish what a given food is. Such definitions are generally long and detailed.
2. Standards of quality: these have been set for a number of foods including canned fruits and vegetables. These are minimum standards only and not grades. FDA may check any food from producer through retailer for its compliance with legal require-

ments for identity, quality, wholesomeness, safety, labeling, and packaging.

3. Standards of fill of container: these require that the container not deceive the consumer with regard to the quantity of food as related to size, shape, or formation of container or to slack fill.

4. Standards for enrichment: these assure the consumer that foods sold as "enriched" actually have had significant amounts of nutrients added and offer guidelines for the processor, the consumer, and the law enforcement agency.

B. Requirements for labeling of foods to prohibit misbranding:

1. The labels for all packaged food must include certain facts which are truthful and not misleading. Information required for different products varies somewhat. For standardized foods, the labels generally need not include a list of ingredients except the presence of any artificial flavoring, coloring, or chemical preservative. Fruit jellies and preserves, butter, and cheddar cheese are examples of such standardized products. Optional ingredients must be listed even for standardized foods.

2. For nonstandardized foods, the major ingredients must be listed on the label in the order of predominance by weight; the nutrient content currently being considered as required information.

3. Food labels must include the name and address of the manufacturer or distributor and an accurate statement of the net amount of food by weight and/or volume in the container.

4. For dietary foods the label must give facts about the dietary properties such as sodium content in "low sodium soups."

5. The required information must be conspicuously displayed and be easy to understand.

C. Prevention of adulteration of food: Adulteration means the process of corrupting, debasing, or making impure "by an admixture of a foreign or baser substance; to prepare, especially for sale, with an ingredient included which is not part of the professed substance, or with an essential ingredient abstracted with a defect artificially concealed or under conditions of exposure to disease, or to simulate a better article."

Adulteration of food is the result of one or more of these conditions:

1. Substitution of some less expensive ingredient is made for a basic ingredient, or the more expensive ingredients are decreased.
2. The addition of substances which are harmful to health occurs, such as unsafe chemical additives, excessive residues of pesticides or antibiotics, or other harmful substances such as decayed items.
3. The addition of filth can occur, such as rodent hair, insect fragments, or other foreign materials which may not be harmful after processing but do violate the esthetic sense of the consumer.

Food additives. According to an FDA statement in 1967, a food additive is any substance put in food that becomes part of the food and/or affects the characteristics of the food. Additives may be intentional when used for some specific purpose, or unintentional when an incidental additive may get into the food while it is grown, processed, packaged, or stored.

Intentional additives may perform one or more of these purposes:
1. To preserve appearance, taste, and wholesomeness such as "antioxidants" which prevent discoloration of fruits and rancidity of fats, or mold inhibitors added to breads and other products.
2. To create and maintain desired consistency of food as emulsifiers that cause tiny food particles to remain uniformly suspended in liquids, and stabilizers which give body, smoothness, and uniformity to a food product.
3. To enhance flavor such as vanilla, monosodiumglutamate, nonnutritive sweeteners, and even spices as salt and pepper.
4. To add nutritive value as in iodized salt, enriched flour, and vitamin A in margarine.
5. To improve color such as dyeing certain oranges, weiners, potatoes, and candies to increase consumer appeal.
6. To perform other functions such as bleaching (make flour look "snowy white" instead of "creamy white"), neutralizing, and buffering.

Common unintentional additives are:
1. Pesticide residues from the spraying of crops or killing of insects and rodents, the fumigation of processing plants, equipment, and storage rooms, or the preservatives used in animal feeds.

2. Drugs as antibiotic residues in milk, meats, and eggs from medicines added to animal feeds or injected into animals to stimulate growth or from veterinary drugs given to animals to prevent or cure disease.
3. Radioactive additives.

Before an intentional additive can be used, it is subjected to toxicity studies by the food and/or chemical manufacturer and is evaluated and regulated by FDA. Toxicity tests are carried on with laboratory animals using amounts of the additive much higher than probably will be ingested by human beings eating the product during a lifetime. Determination of the safety of additives is difficult. Requirements for pre-marketing clearance of additives are that the additive must:

1. perform a useful purpose in the food,
2. be safe for people even if the food were consumed over a lifetime in greater than normal or excessively large amounts, and
3. not contribute to the growth of cancer in laboratory animals even when fed in amounts much greater than will be possible for a person to consume in a lifetime.

The Delaney Amendment to the Food Additive Act of FDA legislation requires that FDA ban any chemical that contributes to the development of any form of cancer in laboratory animals, regardless of the amount of additive required to produce the cancer and how unlikely it would be for any person to consume this amount of the chemical in his whole life.

Pesticide residues in food. If the use of a chemical will leave a residue on food or feed, the chemical cannot be registered until FDA has established a safe tolerance for the residue. The industry or firm promoting the chemical is responsible for obtaining this proof to the satisfaction of FDA which continues its surveillance through additional examination, inspection, and testing of extensive sampling of food products with pesticide residues.

Drug residues on food. More than a thousand pounds of antibiotics are used annually on farms in the United States. Unless drugs are properly administered a certain length of time before the animals are slaughtered, drug residues tend to remain and may endanger the health of people.

Special diet food regulations by FDA. New regulations on special diet foods were published in 1966. The general purpose of the regulation is to give the consumer more facts about the food he buys for reducing body weight and other dietary needs. Such foods are mostly products with reduced sugar or salt content. It has established standards for vitamin and mineral supplements and for foods which may be fortified with these nutrients, this includes accurate labeling.

In spite of these regulations the possibility exists that some of the substances which have been used in the food supply for decades have not been tested adequately. For this reason FDA is committed to restudy the list of substances classed Generally Recognized As Safe, known as the GRAS list, and to continue surveillance of all regulated food additives.

Imported foods. The Bureau of Customs under the Secretary of the Treasury takes the first step in the process of deciding whether a food that comes under the jurisdiction of FDA is admitted or refused entry to this country. Imported food products, the same as domestic ones, are subject to FDA regulations in sampling, examination, and testing before entry as well as in handling, storage, and transportation afterward to insure wholesomeness before entry and freedom from contamination or spoilage after entry.

How the consumer can report to FDA. An FDA "Fact Sheet" suggests what the consumer can do in case he finds a food that is mislabeled,

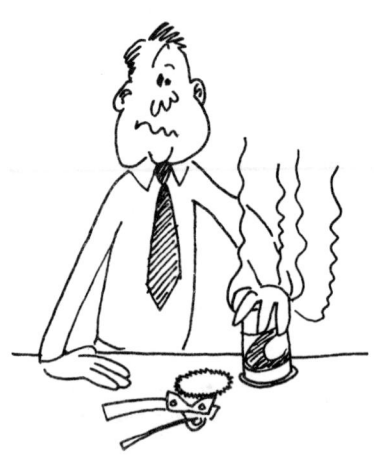

unsanitary, spoiled, or in any way does not comply with the law. First he would report promptly to the merchant the violation or dissatisfaction and have available the product involved, preferably in an unopened container. The consumer and merchant may desire to report to the manufacturer, packer, or distributor of the product. In addition, he can report in writing or by telephone directly to FDA, Department of HEW, Washington, D.C. 20204 or to one of 93 resident inspection stations, which are listed in the telephone directory of that city under U.S. Government, Department of HEW and FDA.

Fig. 10.2 What should the consumer do when he finds food that is unfit for consumption?

The U.S. Department of Agriculture (USDA)

USDA consumer protection is carried on under the Consumer and Marketing Service. This was established as the Agricultural Marketing Service through the 1946 Agricultural Marketing Act and given its present name in 1965. The overall purposes of this act were to provide a scientific approach to the marketing of farm products, an integrated administration of Federal laws resulting in their improved distribution, and "authorized Federal standards for farm products, grading, and inspection services, market expansion activities, consumer education," and related functions.

One of its major responsibilities is underwriting the quality and wholesomeness of much of the nation's food supply through its Consumer Protection programs which include these divisions:

> Compliance Division
> Dairy Products Division
> Division of Fruits and Vegetables
> Livestock Slaughter Inspection Division
> Poultry Division
> Processed Meat Inspection Division
> Technical Services Division

USDA conducts Consumer Food programs which include the School Lunch Division plus various other programs that improve nutrition of school children and provide food primarily for the needy. USDA supports extensive research in food and nutrition as related to increased production and use of agricultural products through the Cooperative Extension Service jointly with the 50 states. The USDA provides a large variety of publications in the form of bulletins, newsletters, research reports, periodicals, and the annual Agricultural Yearbook to furnish useful information for the food consumer. USDA protects the consumer through its food inspection program, which is on a voluntary basis through a fee-for-service trained inspector service for processed fruits and vegetables, but is compulsory for meats. Meats that comply with USDA standards for wholesomeness may be labeled "U.S. Inspected and Passed (Abbreviated: U.S. INSP"D and P'S'D)" plus an inspection number. This label is stamped on fresh meat with safe purple ink and printed on the wrapping or container of processed meat. This is not related to grade, however, only inspected, wholesome meats are graded. Imported foods are passed before entry, after which the same standards apply as for domestic products.

Certificates specifying quality or grade based on USDA Grade Standards (specifications) are available e.g., for canned fruits and vegetables. For fruits, the higher grades (Grade A or Fancy) have greater perfection and uniformity of pieces and a higher concentration of sugar in the juice than the lower grades (Grades B or Choice or Extra Standard and Grade C or Standard). If the quality of the fruit does not meet the degrees of perfection required by the standards, it must be labeled "below standard" or "pie fruit." The fruit may be mushy or in irregular pieces and is canned in water with no added sugar, none of which detract from its wholesomeness.

Nutrient content of different grades of fruits would be comparable except for the increased sugar content of the higher grades contributing to higher calorie value, as is shown in Table 10.1 with data from USDA Handbook No. 8, 1963 revision.

Table 10.1   Energy content in canned fruits.

Fruit and pack		Grade	Calories per 100 grams
Peaches,	water pack	Substandard	31
	light syrup	Standard	58
	heavy syrup	Choice	78
	extra heavy		
	syrup	Fancy	97
Apricots,	water pack	Substandard	38
	light syrup	Standard	66
	heavy syrup	Choice	86
	extra heavy		
	syrup	Fancy	101

Labels for processed fruits and vegetables seldom include grade designations or the fact that they have been processed and packaged under continuous inspection according to USDA standards. Some processors, who use different brand names to designate different grades or quality, do not make this information available to the consumer, however, it can be obtained from the retailer or by writing to the processor.

The Public Health Service (PHS) in the Department of Health, Education, and Welfare (HEW)

The Public Health Service is concerned with the control of food-borne diseases. Early recognition of milk serving as an agent in the transmission of disease led to the development of the Standard Milk Ordinance in 1925. After frequent revision it is now known as "the Grade 'A' Pasteurized Milk Ordinance — 1965 — Recommendations of the U.S. Public Health Service."

PHS has also developed sanitation standards for food service in public eating places, for food and drink vending machines, for poultry processing plants, and for frozen dessert manufacturing. These sanitary standards for all commercial food handlers and for inspection of milk and water are often under the jurisdiction of a sanitarian employed at the local level by a city-county health department.

State and local health departments have the responsibility of administering sanitary regulations and are often in charge of food and drug laws on state and local levels. In this they work closely with representatives from FDA and USDA as well as those from State Departments of Agriculture and of Public Health.

Bureau of Standards — Consumer Protection in Weights and Measures

According to Gordon and Lee (1967), consumers suffer considerable financial loss because of inadequate laws and/or poorly enforced laws regulating weights and measures. In a nationwide survey, state officials who responded to questions in the area of weights and measures estimated that 1–25% of all retailers were deliberately short-weighing products for consumers, with 5% of them doing it most frequently. Also from 10 to 30% with 10% of the retailers doing it most frequently — were "shorting" the customers through carelessness. From 8 to 10% of the measuring devices were found to be inaccurate. Officials from New Jersey and Virginia, which have good laws and enforcement, estimate that "shorting" costs the average family $150 per year. Since weights and measure regulations vary among states and no uniform national law exists, the costs to the consumers vary.

Although the Constitution authorized Congress "to fix the standard of weights and measures," its actions have not been very effective. The question arises, "Would the cost of effective enforcement of weights and measures legislation be an expense or a savings for the consumer of foods?"

The Federal Trade Commission (FTC). This agency, established in 1914, was to combat concentration of excessive economic power through monopolistic practices and to promote fair competition among business enterprises. In 1938, through the Wheeler–Lea Act, FTC had included the protection of the consumer of food, drugs, cosmetics, and therapeutic devices against the dissemination of false or deceptive advertising and other deceptive practices in interstate commerce.

Advertising costs in 1969 approached 20 billion dollars, almost 6% of retail sales, according to The National Industrial Conference Board. The cost for food, confectionery, and beverage advertising in 1968 was first and accounted for 32.6% of all television advertising expenditures. In addition, the food industry that year was first in spot-radio advertising using 20.7% of that budget, third in radio network advertising with 15.0%, and second in newspaper advertising with 13.0%. Advertising for food and beverage corporations was the fourth highest industry and food stores were fifth in money spent for advertising in 1966. In 1969, these food industries were second in amount of advertising and accounted for 18.5% of all advertising expenditures on television.

The 1966 Report of the National Commission on Food Marketing presented advertising costs as a percentage of manufacturers' sales for some selected groceries. These showed a range from vegetable shortening with less than 3%, ready-to-eat cereals with 18%, and powdered coffee whiteners with around 20%. Advertising costs were highest for foods that are recognizably different from traditional foods. The Commission also reported the costs for introducing new food products which could amount to 57% of sales during their first year. "For the average new product preintroductory costs were $68,000 for research and development and $26,000 for market research. Introducing some of these products on a test market basis cost, on the average, an additional $250,000 each." The possible effect of advertising costs of the price of food to the consumer was also reported by the commission as follows:

> In a commission study of 10 such well-established foods as canned peas and frozen orange juice concentrate, retail price of advertised brands averaged 21 per cent higher than retail prices of retailer brands of generally comparable quality.

Although legally, advertising may not make false claims about food, laws do not require that advertising present any specified information about food quality and nutritive value. Nor do laws set any limit on the cost and the kind of promotion which can be used by advertising and selling practices. For example, food markets have long been among the major users of trading stamps, of premiums, and contests to attract customers. Moreover, containers for food may cost as much as their contents and serve as selling aids in addition to protecting the food and facilitating its handling.

Since the primary function of the FTC is to prevent, not punish, it seeks voluntary compliance through its "Trade Practice Conference

Rules," for more than 160 industries. This includes 11 sets of "Advertising Guides." Of course, the FTC may also resort to court action when the voluntary methods do not correct legal violations. Recently the FTC through reorganization formed the Consumer Protection Bureau in order to serve as a major "Consumer Defender's Agency." This includes more emphasis on eliminating deceptive advertising with its earliest attempts directed toward misleading food advertising. New methods for getting compliance with regulations are being explored, such as the recommendation that advertisers provide proof of product claims. Consumers are urged to report fraudulent practices to the FTC.

In addition, the Inspection Service of the U.S. Postal Service is authorized to protect the consumer against fradulent advertising materials sent through the mail. Indirectly, the Federal Communications Commission, FCC, may exercise some control by refusing to issue licenses to radio and television stations that do not operate in the consumer interest: this may include having excessive and/or deceptive advertising.

Consumer Representation in the Office of the President

In 1962, a new kind of recognition was given to the consumer interest of this country when President Kennedy appointed the Consumer Advisory Council (CAC)—a group of 12 private citizens with the Dean of Home Economics, Cornell University, as chairman. It was attached to the Council of Economic Advisers. Its functions were to represent consumers before legislative committees and administrative agencies as well as to keep the President informed of consumer needs and problems.

In 1964, President Johnson expanded consumer representation in the Federal government by establishing the President's Committee on Consumer Interests (PCCI), and appointing a Special Assistant in Consumer Affairs (SACA) to the President. This assistant also served as chairman of PCCI. The 12 member Consumer Advisory Council and high level representatives of 10 government agencies composed PCCI. In addition, Consumer Liaison Officers were appointed by 38 departments and agencies of the Federal government concerned with consumer affairs. The role of PCCI was indicated when President Johnson declared, "I am today taking action to assure that the voice of the consumer will be 'loud, clear, uncompromising, and effective' in the highest councils of the Federal government."

There was an almost immediate response from the public. In the March 1967 report of PCCI the actions were described as follows:

> Mail poured in from every state of the union. In less than a week letters were stacked in the offices of PCCI. Some were written on embossed stationery, some on dime store pads or on the back of package labels. Most had one thing in common—they were written by persons, largely housewives, who had never before corresponded with Government. Many letters were simple expressions of approval.
>
> Comments covered a wide range of problems—prices, packaging, the cost of credit, pesticides, quality, where to address complaints, advertising, care of textiles, appliance repair, product standards, warranties and guarantees, household safety, and nutrition.

Since its establishment, the PCCI and the Special Assistant for Consumer Affairs have been active as spokesman for the consumer interests before government and business and have prepared educational materials, appeared before lay and business groups, conducted conferences, and encouraged the development of consumer groups and programs on state levels. In 1971, the PCCI became the Office of Consumer Affairs.

NONGOVERNMENTAL AND PRIVATE SERVICES FOR THE CONSUMER

Objectives

1. To attend meetings of health and nutrition oriented organizations.
2. To consult with local agencies to improve consumer relationships and meet consumer needs.
3. To demonstrate responsibility for being an informed consumer.

Professional Associations

A number of private agencies are concerned with serving the consumer of food primarily through education instead of legal protection.

The American Dietetic Association (ADA). This organization of professional dietitians has the foremost concern for food and nutrition. Through its journal and other publications, specific conferences, and through the annual national, state, and regional meetings, it strives to keep its membership informed. It cooperates with other organizations, especially those of the health team, to promote nutrition education and to support legislation that would contribute to improved nutrition.

The American Home Economics Association (AHEA). This organization for professional home economists is concerned with the total well-being of the family and its members. Obviously food and nutrition is of importance. The *Journal of Home Economics* includes reports on food and nutrition research and education. AHEA sponsors conferences and programs, in the states and on a national level, for improvement of food labeling, enrichment of food, safety, nutritional needs of children and youth, and related areas.

The American Medical Association (AMA). The largest professional association for medical doctors which through its several journals and conferences tries to keep its membership informed about the health field including nutrition. Through a variety of free and low cost bulletins and leaflets, and the layman's magazine, *Today's Health*, it strives for health education of the public. It cooperates with government agencies such as the FDA to combat food fallacies and frauds through conferences, publication and question and answer service about health products. It is a cosponsor of the Western Hemisphere Nutrition Congress, the third held in August 1971.

Consumer Service Agencies

In order to provide consumers with essential buying information about a variety of consumer goods and services including food, food supplements, and health products, two independent, nonprofit testing laboratories were established: Consumers Research in 1929 and Consumers Union in 1936. Both report their ratings of most of the products which they test on a three-level scale by brand name, explain test methods used, information obtained, and reasons for the rating. Products for testing are obtained through employed buyers who select the products from the retail market the same as any consumer without informing the retailer about the purpose of their purchase. They accept neither advertising for their publications nor permit their test results to be used for advertising by business firms.

Consumers Union claims over a million and a half readers for its magazine, *Consumer Reports*, which includes articles of general interest to consumers in addition to the results of its testing. It has also published a number of books concerned with consumer affairs, conducted consumer education programs, assumed leadership in organizing the International Organization of Consumers Unions (IOCU) and served as spokesman for consumers at hearings held by Federal government agencies.

Consumers Research, which has a much smaller number of subscribers, limits its publication to *Consumer Bulletin* which publishes test results and short discussions about consumer issues. It also participates in hearings of Federal agencies concerned with consumer problems.

Council of Better Business Bureaus was originally organized by a group of businessmen to combat fraudulent advertising. Now it comprises the main organization of business personnel dedicated to keeping business operations fair and honest without government supervision. Operating in the larger cities of every state, Better Business Bureaus protect honest business firms and consumers from the fraudulent practices of the small minority of dishonest ones. Moreover, they provide guidelines through conferences and publication of a variety of bulletins, leaflets, and a book for consumers. In this way they hope to prepare business and consumers to protect themselves and to sell and buy intelligently. Although they do not recommend any business firms or products, they will provide consumers, without cost, information about business firms: usually this information is based on whether the business has received consumer complaints and/or was observed to be deceptive or fraudulent. They encourage consumers who have been cheated by business to file written complaints with the local Better Business Bureau. Although all Better Business Bureaus try to get voluntary compliance with legal and ethical business practices, they will report to the proper legal authorities, business personnel who refuse to comply and cooperate.

In their effort to protect the consumer and to present a favorable image of business, the Better Business Bureaus continue the work against misleading or deceptive advertising. The publication, *A Guide for Retail Advertising and Selling*, in addition to help for retail enterprises, includes guidelines for advertising which are presented as a Fair Practice Code as follows:

1. Serve the public with honest values.
2. Tell the truth about what is offered.
3. Tell the truth in a forthright manner so its significance may be understood by the trusting as well as the analytical individual.
4. Tell customers what they want to know — what they have a right to know and ought to know about what is offered so that they may buy wisely and obtain the maximum satisfaction from their purchases.
5. Be prepared and willing to make good as promised and without quibble on any guarantee offered.
6. Be sure that the normal use of merchandise or services offered will not be hazardous to public health or life.

7. Reveal material facts, the deceptive concealment of which might cause consumers to be misled.
8. Advertise and sell merchandise or service on its merit and refrain from attacking competitors or reflecting unfairly upon their products, services, or methods of doing business.
9. If testimonials are used, use only those of competent witnesses who are sincere and honest in what they say about what is sold.
10. Avoid all tricky devices and schemes such as deceitful trade-in allowances, fictitious list prices, false and exaggerated comparative prices, bait advertising, misleading free offers, and similar practices which prey upon human ignorance and gullibility.

Probably the oldest and best known consumer services used by United States housewives is the Good Housekeeping Seal of Approval. In 1912, William Randolph Hearst, publisher, established the Good Housekeeping Institute, which dealt with household equipment and mechanical devices, and the Good Housekeeping Bureau, which dealt with foods, drugs, and cosmetics. Manufacturers submitted their products for testing without charge; when a manufacturer's product was accepted, i.e., it met Good Housekeeping standards, he was permitted to use the Good Housekeeping Seal of Approval in his advertising and on his labels. According to Gordon and Lee (1967), FTC in 1939 charged Hearst Magazines, Inc., with unfair competition and unfair, deceptive acts and in 1941, issued an order for Good Housekeeping to cease and desist its unfair and deceptive practices. As a result, the Good Housekeeping consumer program was reorganized. The Institute, the Bureau, and the Seal of Approval were discontinued and a single Guaranty Seal was adopted. After some changes, the present oval shaped seal carried this statement: "Good Housekeeping Guarantees – If Product or Performance Defective, Replacement or Refund to Consumer." At present the seal has little significance to the food consumer even though some homemakers and advertisers may think so and imply its assurance of value. Of all the advertisements in the June 1972 issue, only 12 included the seal, and only two advertized food.

The Parents Magazine Seal presents this wording "Refund or Replacement Guaranteed to consumer by *Parents Magazine*; If Product or Performance Is Defective and Reported within 30 days of Purchase." Unlike *Good Housekeeping*, *Parents Magazine* has no testing facilities, but presumably awards the seller the right to use the Seal when his product met *Parent's Magazine's* standards as revealed through tests conducted by a commercial testing company. Gordon and Lee also reported that in

1966 the publisher of *Parents Magazine* agreed to an FTC order prohibiting the magazine from misrepresenting the basis on which its seal was granted. Moreover, the Parents Magazine Seal, the same as Good Housekeeping Guaranty Seal, has been granted to applicants who do a certain amount of advertising with the magazine.

Changing Times is a monthly magazine founded by the Kiplinger Washington Agency in 1947. It includes no advertising and concentrates on a variety of informative articles to assist people with earning and spending money which includes those topics of direct concern to the food consumer. All of the articles are the responsibility of the editorial staff.

The consumers themselves have organized three national voluntary consumer organizations in this country, namely, The National Consumers League (NCL), the American Council on Consumer Interest (ACCI), and the Consumer Federation of America (CFA). The NCL is the oldest, being founded in 1899 to combat undesirable working conditions in sweatshops and child labor. Since then it is committed to legislative action for the consumer.

The American Council on Consumer Interests (ACCI) was organized in 1955 by educators in consumer education with a concern for problems from the viewpoint of the ultimate consumer of goods and services and their need for information. It publishes a newsletter during the nine months of the school year, the semiannual *Journal of Consumer Affairs*, and has added a second newsletter, "The Consumer Education Forum."

The Consumer Federation of America (CFA) was chartered in 1967 and is composed of consumer groups as voting members from city, county, regional, state, and national consumer associations that support CFA objectives and nonvoting group members that are sympathetic to CFA objectives but are not strictly consumer organizations. It publishes the newsletter "Consumer Action."

RESPONSIBILITY OF THE FOOD CONSUMER

All the laws and the work of both government and nongovernment agencies cannot assure the food consumer that his food will be safe, wholesome, and nutritious nor protect him against all economic cheats; he must become intelligently concerned about this protection, make a sincere effort to study and to be informed about his role as consumer so that he can make rational choices in the market place. The apathy to be concerned is the major hurdle in the pursuit of dietary adequacy. Only the individual and the family can decide what they are willing to pay for nutritional benefits and psychological satisfactions.

The three responsibilities of the consumer-buyer of food can be identified as:

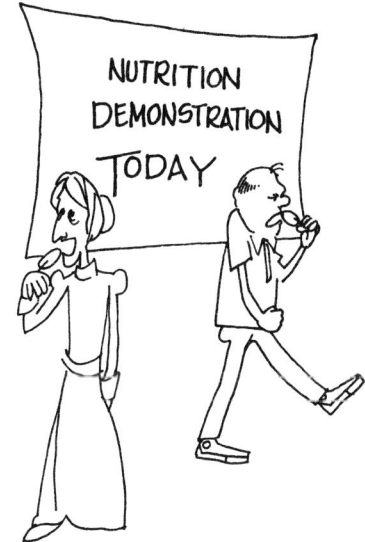

Fig. 10.3 The apathy to be concerned is a major hurdle in the pursuit of dietary adequacy.

1. The consumer as purchasing agent for himself and the family: since the majority of the United States families buy most of their food instead of producing it at home, the food buyer largely determines the family diet, and consequently, its nutrient content, the value received for the food dollar, and the extent of food waste in the home. To protect the health of the family and to get a fair return for the money spent for food, the food buyer must be informed and concerned about these factors:

   (a) Nutritive needs and food preferences of family members. Food should provide both essential nutrients and enjoyment. Food should serve physiological as well as psychological and social needs of individuals and families.

   (b) The nutritive value and comparative costs of the edible portions of various foods as well as the amounts appropriate in volume and nutrient content for different family members at meals and for snacks are the responsibility of the homemaker. This will enable him to get the best return both nutritionally and financially for money spent through effective consumer buying and meal planning.

   (c) The proper methods of storing, preparing, and serving of different foods in order to conserve nutrients, enhance appetite appeal, and minimize waste of food, money, time, and energy are required. This includes selecting quality on the basis of intended use.

   (d) Ways of keeping mealtime pleasant through a relaxed atmosphere in comfortable, attractive surroundings are vital.

Tensions and strong negative emotions such as worry, anger, hate, frustration, and fear can counteract the benefits of even the most nutritional and appetizing meal.

(e) The psychology underlying food preferences, dislikes, choices, and dietary habits must be understood in order to guide family members, particularly children, to develop sound eating habits.

2. The consumer as a customer of business: the food buyer can serve himself and other consumers best by following these guidelines:

(a) Deal only with ethical business firms.

(b) Inform business personnel of what she approves and what she would like in food products sold, facilities and services provided, and business methods used as the result of study, thinking and concern for the common good.

If the consumer disapproves of a business firm to the extent that he will no longer patronize it, he should give the firm his reasons for discontinuing this relationship.

(c) Understand the overall reasons for food prices and to be aware that in the United States economy everyone involved in the production and distribution of food is entitled to a fair income. For example, convenience foods, with a few exceptions, are more expensive in monetary cost but less expensive in time, energy, and facility costs than foods which require more preparation. Likewise, extensive advertising, elaborate facilities, many customer services, and promotional gimmicks as trading stamps, contests, premiums, and fancy packaging cost money.

(d) The extent to which the consumer may add to food prices varies with the situation. To be an honest considerate consumer-buyer who does not abuse merchandise, facilities, or services is essential. All destructive and dishonest practices such as shoplifting and vandalism by

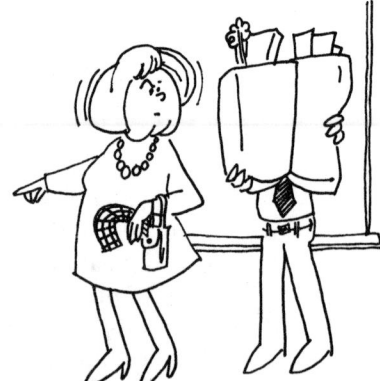

Fig. 10.4 Consumers wonder about food prices while they demand more services, premiums, and trading stamps.

employees, customers, and their children add to costs of operating the business and eventually results in higher prices. Recent magazine articles have reported that some merchants have to raise prices 15% to compensate for shoplifting losses.

3. Consumer citizenship which includes the following:
   (a) Supporting government and private agencies that are effective in consumer protection and/or education.
   (b) Promoting needed laws and programs for consumer well-being, opposing those not needed, those that are too expensive for services provided, that curb individual freedom excessively, and/or that favor only a small group at the expense of the majority.
   (c) Voting for governmental candidates who are prepared for the office and are ethical in performing their work. Voting without being informed about the candidate, the issues, or the program may be more detrimental to the country than not voting at all.
   (d) Being an ethical, intelligent consumer-citizen whose citizenship responsibilities increase in significance as scientific-technological-social-economic conditions make it necessary for government to perform more services for its people, services that would not be profitable for private enterprise and regulatory-protective responsibilities that individuals cannot provide for themselves.

      When individuals and business do not solve problems facing them, government will, and thus relieve them of their own initiative and of some freedom.

      Only through responsible action of all areas of the food industry and of the majority of food consumers will the need for more government regulations be minimized and essential regulations made more effective.

Activities for Student Learning

A. Consider yourself as a consumer who is concerned about acquiring an adequate diet to achieve optimum nutrition. What would be your recommendations in these situations? You may wish to role-play these problems and have classmates portray the different viewpoints and professional positions.

   1. Survey the food marketing situation in your locale and in some which differ greatly from yours (affluent in contrast to poverty areas).

    (a) Note differences in marketing practices and try to identify the reasons; consultation with the store manager would be essential.

    (b) Note problems in merchandizing food which these businesses have in common.

2. Study and visit with consumers in each neighborhood and in different types of stores to ascertain their similarities and differences of attitude, behavior, and needs.

3. Observe the consumer food buyer in action without his being aware of your observing him. Note to what extent he reads the labels.

4. If feasible, prepare a simple questionnaire that would reveal the knowledge and perhaps the attitudes toward their protection as a food consumer. You need to ask for permission from the manager of the business and of the customers for you to administer the questionnaire. Be sure to explain the objectives for wanting this information. Tabulate data, analyze, draw conclusions, and evaluate.

    You could use a food business catering to university students.

5. What references to consumer practices did you note in literature which you have read?

6. Don't forget!

Hot Tips:

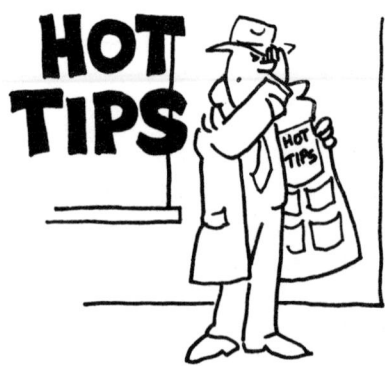

New Words:

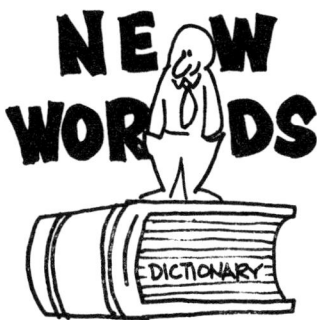

B. In general we need to acquaint ourselves with local facilities and services which are concerned about the consumer being given a "square deal" or a fair chance.

  1. Visit and interview selected personnel of a private consumer services and include such items as:
    (a) Become acquainted with the purposes or functions of the agency, how its responsibilities are performed, and the greatest needs for its work.
    (b) If it has publications for the consumer, become acquainted with them and determine their possible value to the food consumer.
    (c) Learn what the individuals think consumers can and should do to protect themselves and assist this agency.
    (d) Draw conclusions and evaluate your experience.
  2. Also visit and interview a business concerned with food.
    (a) Visit the firm to learn from its manager about its efforts to serve and please the consumer.
    (b) Get opinions of personnel with regard to consumer protection laws under which the business is operating. How readily can a business comply with these laws? What are the costs involved?
    (c) Learn opinion of personnel with regard to the attitudes and behavior of the consumers they serve — their customers. How do they make it easy or difficult — even costly — for the business to serve them?

(d) What do they wish customers would know and do or not do when they patronize this business?
3. Collect a variety of labels from food packages, analyze and classify them according to their use as buying aids. Explain which ones comply with the legal requirements, which ones seem questionable, and which ones give inadequate information for an intelligent consumer choice.

What additional information would you recommend? Please support your opinions with facts and reasons.

C. Procedure for conducting a consumer survey: To conduct a reliable consumer survey a systematic procedure needs to be followed which includes a logical sequence of events.
1. *Objectives* — determine purposes to be achieved:
   (a) What are you trying to prove or find out about a certain product or a consumer practice?
   (b) Will you compare brand names, quality, cost, palatability, preparation time, nutritive value, particularly in relation to cost?
2. *Procedure* — establish a sequence of events to solve the problem:
   (a) How will this study be conducted?
   (b) How will you make *valid* comparisons, etc.?
   (c) Did you have references to help you decide on methodology?
3. *Results and Discussion*
   (a) You may use graphs, charts, labels, etc. with which to compare findings.
   (b) Present results in a concise manner, preferably in a table with proper design and in a graph correctly executed.
4. *Conclusions and recommendations*
   (a) Will you make any changes in your buying habits as a result of your study?
   (b) What do you recommend in relation to objectives?
   (c) Will you influence other consumers in making better decisions?

Invite representatives from different areas of the food industry, consumer service organizations, and of government to present their viewpoints, their efforts, and problems in providing wholesome nutritious food for the consumer.

Develop a composition which is suitable for publication in a lay publication such as *Today's Health* on some aspect of the subject, "The U.S. Consumer Assumes Responsibility for His Own Nutritional Status."

Selected References and Suggested Readings

A Guide for Retail Advertising and Selling, 6th ed. (rev.) Assoc. of Better Business Bureaus, Inc., New York, 1963.

A Summary of Activities (1964–1967), President's Committee on Consumer Interests, Washington, D.C., 1967.

Biesdorf, H. B., and Burris, M. E. *Be A Better Shopper: Buying in the supermarkets.* Ithaca, N.Y.: Cornell University, 1968.

Consumer Education Bibliography, Office of Consumer Affairs, Executive Office of the President, U.S. Govt. Ptg. Office, Washington, D.C., 1971.

Consumer Information, U.S. Govt. Ptg. Office, Washington, D.C.

Consumer Protection Activities of State Governments – Part 2 – The Regulation of Foods and Related Products, Seventh Report of the Committee of Government Operations, U.S. Govt. Ptg. Office, Washington, D.C., 1963.

Consumers All, The Yearbook of Agriculture, Washington, D.C., Supt. Doc., 1965.

Cross, J. *The Supermarket Trap* (the consumer and the food industry), Indiana University Press, Bloomington, Inc., 1970.

Food for Us All, The Yearbook of Agriculture, Washington, D.C., Supt. Doc., 1969.

Food from Farmer to Consumer, Report of the National Commission on Food Marketing, U.S. Govt. Ptg. Office, Washington, D.C., 1966.

Gordon, L. J., and Lee, S. M. *Economics for Consumers*, 6th ed. New York: Amer. Book Co., 1972.

Guide to Federal Consumer Services, Office of Consumer Affairs, Executive Office of the President, U.S. Govt. Ptg. Office, Washington, D.C., 1971.

Kinder, F. *Meal Management*, 3rd ed. New York: Macmillan, 1968.

Money Management, Your Food Dollar, 1970, Your Shopping Dollar, 1969. Money Management, Institute, Household Finance Corporation, Chicago, 1970.

Protecting Our Food, The Yearbook of Agriculture, Washington, D.C., Supt. Doc., 1966.

Troelstrup, A. W. *The Consumer in American Society*, 4th ed. New York: McGraw-Hill, 1970.

Periodicals

A watchdog growls – Federal Trade Agency sets out to prove it is the consumer's friend, *Wall Street J.*, **47**: 37, 1 (1971).

Bauman, H. E. Nutrient labeling – purpose and approach, *Food Tech.*, **25**: 611, 47 (1971).

Cabinet rank for us shoppers?, *Changing Times*, **23**: 6, 15 (1969).

Clements, F. W., Conflict in nutrition – commerce versus consumers, *Food & Nutr. Notes & Rev.*, **27**, 109 (1970).

Coltrin, D. M., and Bradfield, R. B. Food buying practices of urban low-income consumers – a review, *J. Nutr. Educ.*, **1**: 3, 16 (1970).

Coon, J. M. Naturally occurring toxicants in foods, *Food Tech.*, **23**, 104 (August 1969).

Got a gripe? Here's where to complain, *Changing Times*, **24**: 3, 31 (1970).

MacGregor, J. Heavy thumbs – short-weighting often leaves consumer paying more for less, *Wall Street J.*, **48**: 2, 1 (1971).

McFarlane, A. N. Of convenience, food innovation and calling the tune: The revolutionary imperative, *Food Tech.*, **23**, 43 (1969).

Mead, M., The changing significance of food, *The Amer. Sci.*, **58**, 176 (1970).

Meat inspection – notice of proposed rule making, *Fed. Registrar*, **34**, 1394 (1969).

Melnick, D. Development of organoleptically and nutritionally improved margarine products, *J. Home Eco.*, **60**, 793 (1968).

Sanders, H. J. Food additives, Parts I & II, *Chem. & Engn. News*, **44**, 100 and 108 (1966).

Standal, B. R., Bassett, D. R., Policar, P. B., and Thom, M. Fatty acids, cholesterol, and proximate analysis of some ready-to-eat foods, *J. Amer. Dietet. Assoc.*, **56**, 392 (1970).

Stavenger, P., The food industry and pollution, *Food Tech.*, **24**, 121 (February 1970).

Substitute milk, *Consumer Reports*, **34**, 8 (1969).

The great White House hope—report on the Conference on Food, Nutrition and Health, *Food Tech.*, **24**, 100 (1970).

Vickery, J. R. Possible developments in the supply and utilization of food in the next 50 years, *Food Tech.*, **25**: 619, 55 (1971).

What's happened to truth-in-packaging?, *Consumer Reports*, **34**, 40 (1969).

FDA Publications

Additives in Our Food, FDA's Life Protection Series, 1969.

FDA Fact Sheet:

    Enforcing the Food, Drug, and Cosmetic Act, CSS, G6, 1968.

    Food Standards, 9, 1968.

    How the Consumers Can Report to FDA, CSS, G3, 269.

    Quackery, 486.

    Special Dietary Regulations, 1967.

Requirements of the U.S. Food, Drug, and Cosmetic Act, FDA Publ. No. 2, revised 1967.

Significant Dates in Food and Drug Law History, FDA Publ. No. 20, 1968.

FDA Papers

Certified shellfish, **3**: 4, 8 (1969).

Cook, J. W. Pesticide Multiresidue Methodology (finding multiresidues on foods), **2**: 9, 4 (1968).

Duggan, R. E. Controlling Aflotoxins, **4**: 3, 13 (1970).

Duggan, R. E., and Dawson, K. Pesticides—a report on residues in food, **1**: 5, 1 (1967).

FDA units and their functions, **4**: 4, 4 (1970).

Fischback, H. Industrial chemicals and FDA, **4**: 7, 8 (1970).

Gomez, L. M. Food and drug imports, **2**: 3, 16 (1968).

Heath, G. E. Customs and FDA, **2**: 3, 4 (1968).

Labonski, A. Single system, multiple benefits, **4**: 9, 13 (1970).

Lindsay, D. R. Food safety, **4**: 6, 4 (1970).

Olson, J. C. Microbiological food hazards and regulatory control, **2**: 10, 4 (1968).

Silverman, M., Consumer education and information, **30**: 2, 4 (1971).

Simmons, S. W. Living labs that study how pesticides affect man, **3**: 4, 13 (1969).

Slomoff, R. J., and Freerer, R. E., Jr. FDA-FTC Liason: Teamwork that pays off, **30**: 3, 4 (1971).

Spiher, A. T. The GRAS list review, **4**: 10, 12 (1971).

Van Howeling, C. D. Use of antibiotics in food animals: A review and status report, **3**: 4, 21 (1969).

USDA Publications

A Consumer's Guide to USDA Services, Misc. Publ. No. 959, U.S. Govt. Ptg. Office, Washington, D.C., 1968.

Available Publications of USDA's Consumer and Marketing Service, C & MS 53, USDA, 1971.

Gale, H. F. Outlook for food prices, consumption, and expenditures, Statement made to National Agricultural Outlook Conference, USDA, 1971.

Meat, fish, poultry, and cheese: Home preparation time, yield, and composition of various market forms, Home Eco. Research Report No. 30, ARS, USDA, 1965.

Peterkin, B., and Cromwell, C. Convenience and the cost of food, Family Eco. Rev., ARS 62–65, USDA 9 (June 1971).

Standards for meat and poultry products—a consumer reference list, C & MS, USDA, 1971.

USDA Grade Names—for food and farm products, C & MS 69, USDA, 1969.

INVENTORY OF KNOWLEDGE
Part I   Matching

A. Match the advertising or labeling information with its meaning for the consumer:

_____ 1. USDA Large Grade A eggs

_____ 2. Vita-rich bread — so rich in vitamins it will make you look and feel younger

Consumer information

(a) provides specific useful information
(b) is largely meaningless
(c) is misleading or false

_____ 3. This sausage is guaranteed to be the best quality

_____ 4. Pure strawberry preserves

_____ 5. Lose weight the Easy Way with Slimesterole—a secret reducing formula to be eaten with your regular meals.

_____ 6. Use our fruit drink daily for a beautifully healthy complexion

_____ 7. This flour is enriched 12 different ways!

_____ 8. All-beef wieners are a nutritious treat.

_____ 9. Made for the nutrition conscious mother.

_____ 10. Picnic hams are labeled "water added."

B. Match the services with the agency that performs it.

_____ 11. Protects the consumer against deceptive advertising of food

_____ 12. Discusses and often rates foods by brand name according to tests and study

(a) USDA
(b) FDA
(c) BBB
(d) FTC
(e) Consumers Union
(f) Postal Inspection Service

_____ 13. Sets standards of identity and quality for certain foods

_____ 14. Checks meats for wholesomeness

_____ 15. Protects consumer against deceptive and fraudulent advertisements sent through the mail

_____ 16. Is in charge of the enrichment of bread and flour

_____ 17. Gives information on a local sales representative

_____ 18. Identifies adulteration in food

_____ 19. Specifies requirements of Type A school lunch

_____ 20. Determines if advertising is deceptive

Part II   Choose the Single Correct Answer

21. Check the statement that is *not* true about the services of FDA:
    (a) sets standards of identity for foods
    (b) checks that food labeling meets legal requirements and is not misleading
    (c) is responsible for the grading of fruits and vegetables
    (d) protects against adulteration of foods
    (e) tries to prevent misleading packaging and slack fill of containers

22. Check statement that is not true about USDA services:
    (a) inspection of meats and poultry for wholesomeness
    (b) compulsory grading of all meats and poultry in interstate commerce
    (c) publication of a variety of educational bulletins, newsletters, and periodicals
    (d) setting standards for grading of agricultural products including fruits and vegetables
    (e) Cooperative Extension Service is involved in teaching

Part III   True – False

Mark the entirely true statements with plus (+) and those not true with minus (–) and support your decision when needed:

_____ 23. A close relationship exists between nutrient content and price of food.

_____ 24. Wholesome food contains no chemicals.

_____ 25. Some consumer practices and demands add to the cost of retailing food thus contributing to higher prices.

_____ 26. Major large food corporations have among the highest advertising expenditures among United States industries.

_____ 27. The family that wants to maximize the return on its food expenditures will serve bacon (95¢ a pound) instead of ham ($1.69 per pound) for breakfast.

____ 28. Information about the grades and standards for meats and meat products can be obtained from USDA.

____ 29. Food bought in larger quantities or containers always costs less per serving than the same food bought in smaller quantities.

____ 30. Generally, Federal Government Agencies have jurisdiction only over products and business practices in interstate commerce.

____ 31. All kinds of consumer complaints may be addressed to the Office of Consumer Affairs in the Executive Office of the President.

____ 32. The higher grades of food, such as those of beef and canned fruits, assure the consumer a superior nutrient supply to that in lower grades.

____ 33. Food likes and dislikes are formed early in life.

____ 34. Because food additives tend to be harmful to the health of people they should all be banned.

____ 35. A major responsibility of FDA is to check that pesticide and drug residues in food are within safe limits.

____ 36. The consumer is assured of a bargain whenever she buys a high grade of food at below its regular price.

____ 37. A product labeled "Pure Maple Syrup" may contain only a small amount of cane sugar.

____ 38. If adequate consumer protection laws were passed and effectively enforced, every United States citizen would be well nourished.

____ 39. Cereal in package with net weight of 18 oz selling for 77 cents costs less per ounce than the same cereal sold in a package of 13 oz for 53 cents.

____ 40. The term, net weight, on a food package means the weight of the contents plus that of the container.

____ 41. Both the first Federal Food and Drug Act and the Meat Inspection Act were passed in the same year, 1906.

____ 42. The Delaney Clause, as a part of the Food Additive Amendment, sets standards too low to protect the consumer against cancer.

____ 43. Consumer protection responsibilities are divided among a large number of Federal Government Agencies.

____ 44. Only when nutrient content and quality of food are described in standardized terms on the label can the consumer make valid comparisons in purchasing packaged food.

_____ 45. Protection for the food buyer varies greatly on state and local levels among the 50 states.

_____ 46. In this country only the very low income individuals lack a nutritionally adequate diet.

_____ 47. The national weights and measures law assures the consumer that the Bureau of Standards prevents short-weighing of food packages.

_____ 48. The government should take full responsibility in the protection of nutritional welfare of the consumer.

_____ 49. Basically food in the United States is produced by reliable agriculture and processed, stored, and sold by responsible industry and business.

_____ 50. The consumer needs to assume responsibility to be informed, to know where to get reliable information, and to try to keep abreast of change.

Part IV

Students should look for current news releases about the developments in the Federal regulations of nutrition information in food labeling and in open-dating and unit pricing of food. Make a survey to determine the consumer's use of these informational labeling regulations. Identify the information needed by consumers to utilize the information released by the FDA.

Finis

What does human nutrition mean? Does it mean a vital force available through pleasant and exciting food from an agricultural and industrial abundance? Today a status of nutritional achievement is available to every person who takes advantage of the facilities and opportunities around him. True, every person is not born equal; nevertheless, food supplies are of high quality and in relatively great abundance such as the world has not previously known. Obviously, in the world food per capita is inadequate to meet either the optimum biological needs of every person or the eccentricities of his food acceptance. Neither the efficiency of production and capacity for food processing, storage, and distribution, nor the awareness of the need for population control have been applied to man's problems of survival.

Why is nutrition information accepted so slowly by otherwise know-ledgeable people? Why does man continue to look for magical easy solutions to his dietary problems? Why does he not practice those rational behaviors that contribute to good health? To be concerned about vast populations in distant lands is commendable; their plight is truly desperate in many areas, especially when natural catastrophies are added to man's irrational actions. But what about the individual in an affluent society? Has he performed and lived today based on the information gained through the study of nutrition? Knowledge written in a book unread or ignored is like music which was played but unheard. Does either really exist?

Yesterday needs to be the deadline for malnutrition and the prolog for nutrition education; *Today* is the time for all-out effort to alleviate hunger, indifference, and ignorance about food and dietary practices and the existence of *Tomorrow* is dependent on the success of *Today*. An excellent summary is presented in the quotation by Lillian Storms Coover, former president of The American Dietetic Association:

> For Yesterday is but a Dream
> And Tomorrow but a Vision
> But Today well lived makes
> Every Yesterday a Dream of Happiness
> And Every Tomorrow a Vision of Hope.

Appendixes

A COMMON SYMBOLS FOR USE IN NUTRITION EDUCATION

ADA	American Dietetic Association
AID	Agency for International Development
CSM	Corn, Soya, and Milk (mix for adequate nutrient supply)
DNA	Deoxyribonucleic Acid
FAO	Food and Agriculture Organization of the United Nations
FPC	Fish Protein Concentrate
ICNND	Interagency Committee on Nutrition for National Defense
INCAP	Institute for Nutrition in Central America and Panama
INCAPARINA	Plant-protein blend developed by INCAP
IU	International Unit
NRC	National Research Council
PER	Protein Efficiency Rate
P/S	Polyunsaturated fats ratio to Saturated fats
RDA	Recommended Daily Allowance
RNA	Ribonucleic Acid
UNESCO	United Nations Educational, Scientific, and Cultural Organization
UNICEF	United Nations Children's Fund
USDA	United States Department of Agriculture
USHEW	United States Department of Health, Education, and Welfare
USP	United States Pharmacopia
WHO	World Health Organization of the United Nations

B   ANSWERS TO INVENTORY OF KNOWLEDGE

Section 2   Basic Concepts of Human Nutrition

Part I

A.	1. c	B.	9. b
	2. b		10. a
	3. b		11. d
	4. f		12. f
	5. c		13. g
	6. d		14. b
	7. e		15. c
	8. d		16. e

Part II

17. all of these
18. all of these
19. a
20. b
21. d
22. b, d, c, e
23. a

Section 3   Growth and Development as Indicators of Nutritional Status

Part I

1. nutrition
2. skull; brain
3. anterior-posterior; skeleton; carpal bones, wrist
4. designer; nutrition; dietetics
5. iron; ascorbic acid
6. food; education; contamination, infection, or parasites

Part II

7. d
8. a
9. e
10. a, b, c, e
11. a, b, c, d
12. a, b, c
13. e

Part III

14. a, d	19. e (or any)
15. a, b	20. e or any one
16. a, e	21. e or any
17. b, e	22. c
18. b, c	23. d ($\frac{1}{2}$ lb lost per week)

24. anemic, apathetic, weak, phlegmatic, distended stomach, edematus, listless, emaciated, tired, pale, fatigued, fears, super-stitions, rejection, skeletal malalignment

Section 4   Dietary Specifications to Meet Nutritional Needs

Part I

1. T	7. T
2. T	8. F
3. T	9. T
4. F	10. F
5. T	11. T but bread is questionable
6. T	

12. T This depends on the type structure of vegetable, size of pieces, whole or cut, etc.
13. T & F depending on age group, health, and socioeconomic condition

Part II

14. a	17. b	20. b
15. a	18. d	
16. d	19. c	

Section 5   The Body's Need for Nutrients: Dietary Supply

Part I

1. c	5. e or any
2. a	6. b
3. a	7. c
4. d	8. d

Part II

		calories
9. (a)	4 oz orange juice	29
	1 fried egg (1 T fat)	180
	3 strips of crisp bacon	135
	1 slice toast	70
	$\frac{1}{2}$ T butter on toast	50
	$\frac{1}{2}$ C skimmed milk	45

509 calories in breakfast

(b) Of 2000 calories daily energy expenditure, 500–667 calories should be consumed at breakfast. This breakfast, which furnishes 509 calories is sufficient for this person.

10. Check discussion given in this section.

Section 7   Protein as a Source of Amino Acids

Part I

1. e	4. a	7. c
2. c	5. a	
3. a	6. e	

Part II

8. Amino acid supplementation means that one amino acid may be added to a diet which contains food low in that amino. acid. For example, corn is very low in lysine but a diet in which the protein supply is dependent on corn, can be supplemented with lysine in correct amount and achieve a high biological value.

9. One food which is abundant in an amino acid may serve to supplement a deficient amount in another food, as for example: milk proteins which are low in methionine and high in lysine content would make an excellent supplement to cereal proteins which are very low in lysine, but generous in the concentration of methionine.

10. Early signs of protein deficiency in college-age women could be irregular and limited menstruation, chronic fatigue (when sleep is adequate), pallor, listlessness, apathy.
11. The method used to describe the procedure to establish the biological value of a protein consists of feeding standard test animals a ration adequate in all respects except for the amount of protein.
12. Limiting amino acid refers to that amino acid which first is in insufficient amount when the protein is fed at some practical level in the diet. The first limiting amino acids in corn and other cereals is lysine.
13. Meats, milk, and eggs (the protein foods) supply the highest portion of the protein intake of families. The daily amount is easily furnished by 4 oz EP meat, 1 pt to 1 qt milk and 1 egg.
14. The proteolytic enzymes are as follows: stomach — gastric proteinase or pepsin; small intestine — trypsin and erepsin
15. Lysosomes of the cell contain enzymes which degradate protein molecules.
16. First step in the metabolism of amino acids is the peptide bond formation between the amine group of one amino acid and the carboxyl of another to form dipeptides.
17. The DNA has the code for the sequence of peptide linkages required in the protein synthesis of a cell. This sequence is transmitted by an RNA molecule to the robosome where enzymes have lined up the individual amino acids for linking.
18. 1 egg; $48 \text{ g} \times 12\%$ protein   5.76
    2 sl. toast; $50 \text{ g} \times 8\%$ protein   4.00
    1 glass milk; $224 \text{ g} \times 3.5\%$ protein   7.84
    ⎯⎯⎯⎯⎯⎯⎯⎯
    17.60 g total protein

    RDA for 55 kg woman = 49.5 g; $\frac{17.6}{49.5} \times 100 = 35.5\%$ of RDA

Section 8   Mineral Elements in Human Nutrition

Part I

1. b	10. b	19. a
2. e	11. b	20. b
3. b	12. b	21. f
4. e	13. b	22. a, c, f
5. b	14. d	23. e
6. b	15. a	24. b
7. a	16. d	25. a
8. a	17. b	
9. c	18. f	

Part II	29. e
26. a	30. e
27. a	31. a
28. e	32. c

33. Mineral elements are released from their structural and chemical involvement in the food and made soluble in the gastro-intestinal fluids by the action of digestive enzymes on carbohydrates, fats, and proteins.
34. T
35. See objective 3, page 193.
36. T
37. Most women's diets are deficient in iron. The average 1000 calories in a given diet contribute about 6 mg of iron.
38. Technology supplies excess sodium through additives and residues in food.
39. T
40. T
41. Calcium is the most abundant mineral element in the human body.
42. T
43. T
44. Thyroxine contains iodine in its molecular structure.
45. T

Section 9 Vitamins in Human Nutrition

Part I

1. e	10. e	18. d
2. b	11. c	19. f
3. c	12. b	20. b
4. b	13. e	21. b
5. f	14. a	22. a
6. d	15. d	23. b
7. c	16. a	24. f
8. g	17. a	25. a
9. b		

Part II

26. Discovery of vitamins was due to:
    (a) limited, seasonal food supplies
    (b) limited supply of food during long voyages or trips
    (c) processing of the major food such as rice
    (d) inadequate storage of perishable foods both plant and animal
    (e) limited food acceptability
    (f) curiosity of thoughtful people in trying to identify causes of illnesses
27. Vitamins function as:
    (a) enzyme-type catalysts
    (b) production and maintenance of certain tissues
    (c) indispensable to growth and life
    (d) required for physical and mental health

28. Reduction of vitamin content in food may be attributed to:
    (a) varietal differences in species of plants and in different stages of maturity
    (b) wilting and deterioration during storage especially at temperatures above 50°F
    (c) leaching during washing, blanching, or cooking
    (d) cooked too long, cut into too small pieces
    (e) excessive exposure to air, especially at higher temperatures
    (f) delayed eating after preparation
29. Vitamin supplements should be selected on basis of
    (a) deficiency of diet
    (b) single or multiple deficiency symptoms
    (c) type of bodily dysfunction
    (d) cost of various brand name of comparable composition
    (e) potency of tablet related to need

Section 10   The Concern of the Consumer for Food and Nutrition

Part I			Part II	Part III			
A.	1. a	B. 11. d	21. c	23. false	32. false	41. true
	2. c	12. e	22. b	24. false	33. true	42. false
	3. b	13. b		25. true	34. false	43. true
	4. a	14. a		26. true	35. true	44. true
	5. c	15. f		27. false	36. false	45. true
	6. c	16. b		28. true	37. false	46. false
	7. c	17. c		29. false	38. false	47. false
	8. a	18. b		30. true	39. false	48. false
	9. b	19. a		31. true	40. false	49. true
	10. a	20. d				50. true

C SYMBOLS FOR SOME CHEMICAL ELEMENTS USED IN NUTRITION

Ag	Silver	Hg	Mercury
Al	Aluminum	I	Iodine
Au	Gold	K	Potassium
B	Boron	Mg	Magnesium
Ba	Barium	Mn	Manganese
C	Carbon	Mo	Molybdenum
Ca	Calcium	N	Nitrogen
Cd	Cadmium	Na	Sodium

Cl	Chlorine	O	Oxygen
Co	Cobalt	P	Phosphorus
Cu	Copper	Pb	Lead
F	Fluorine	S	Sulfur
Fe	Iron	Se	Selenium
H	Hydrogen	Zn	Zinc
He	Helium		

Index